Neuroliterature 3
Biography, Semiology, Miscellany

More perspectives on the nervous system and its disorders

AJ LARNER

AJ Larner MD DHMSA PhD FRCP(UK)

Consultant Neurologist, Walton Centre for Neurology and Neurosurgery, Liverpool, L9 7LJ, United Kingdom

Formerly Society of Apothecaries' Honorary Lecturer in the History of Medicine, University of Liverpool, United Kingdom.

e-mail: ajlarner241@aol.com

THE CHOIR PRESS

First published in the United Kingdom in 2025 by
The Choir Press

ISBN 978–1–78963–529–4

Contents

Foreword

The author of this book, Andrew Larner, is a clinical neurologist with thirty years' experience and with a particular interest in and knowledge of cognitive neurology. He is therefore well placed to bring to all of us writings and analysis of the work of others in medical history and thus the contributions here cover a wide range in the field of history. He also explains his decision to relinquish clinical medicine in favour of medical history and, although he is not the first to do this, he is the most recent and accomplished in the field. He has published widely in Liverpool where he has worked, and in journals in many other domains and has edited the *Journal of Medical Biography* with a wide choice of original papers from authors around the world, not only in the neurological field but in many areas. That journal was founded by the Royal Society of Medicine in London in order to record the contributions of those whose lives would not otherwise have been recorded and therefore many not initially well-known persons have come to our knowledge and helped guide us in the development of medicine to help us try to help others.

Biography is a mainstay of the history of medicine and so popular since the study of our fellow human beings throws so much light on what we have done and what we hope to do. Thus in this book we find vignettes and longer pieces about other authors and in other disciplines and all of this should provide a great deal of interesting reading for many persons. As Alexander Pope reminded us, the proper study of mankind is man.

Here we find not only biography but many other aspects of medical history including places and all sorts of developments but in addition copious ideas and analyses. What sort of procedures in the mind of each of us can allow a wealth of memories from copious reading? Some say the brain works like a computer. We would have to ask how on earth it does work and the answer surely is not by analogy with our own inventions including powerful computing machines.

The reader will need to decide whether to absorb this book from start to finish, as this writer did, or whether to dip into the areas of particular interest to him or her. Each method obviously is fine but it will be wise not to miss out any of the jewels to be found in these pages. This should provide not only knowledge and learning but also delight in many areas that are not well covered elsewhere.

We are told that this volume is the final of three volumes that together provide a trilogy in neurological history writing, but the knowledge that the author is leaving clinical medicine to work in history must surely provide a great deal of hope that much more similar literature will emerge in the coming months and years.

Christopher Gardner-Thorpe
Exeter UK

Introduction

In this final volume of *Neuroliterature*, complementing the earlier volumes (2019, 2023), it is perhaps pertinent to ask whether these divertimenti serve any purpose? The unanswered question (Charles Ives)! Some topics are worked through fairly thoroughly, some are little more than promptings for further research, some merely musings. My semantic space is broad, but not necessarily deep! All have engaged me at one time or another over the past 40 years, and it is my hope that some might similarly engage readers of this volume.

Biography

Goldsmith ... described the biography as "the most useful manner of writing, not only from the pleasure it affords the imagination, but from the instruction it artfully and unexpectedly conveys to the understanding".

Coote S (ed.). *Oliver Goldsmith. The Vicar of Wakefield.* London: Penguin Classics, 1986:10–11

Further thoughts on medical biography

1. Medical biography: a symbiotic methodology?

In his recent [2023] *Journal of Medical Biography* editorial, Henry Connor recommended Rudyard Kipling's six honest serving men – What, Why, When, How, Where, and Who – as guides to the writing of medical biography.[1] These questions – with the exception of Who – also underpin the first step of the "Systemizing Mechanism" postulated by Simon Baron-Cohen to underlie the human capacity for invention,[2] a capacity undoubtedly also necessary for writing biography. Kipling's serving men also stood as the epigraph to a book which contributed to my basic medical training in clinical history taking,[3] and I have advocated summoning them in the context of assessing patients with symptoms of impaired memory.[4] Hence, I am sympathetic to Henry Connor's recommendations. Nevertheless, I suggest that some further qualification is necessary, and that a different model, ultimately derived from the biological sciences, might better serve medical biography, at least in some instances.

The problem with the "Kipling approach" is that the sheer number of potential Whats, Whys, Whens, Hows, Wheres, and Whos in any life is likely to be daunting, and many will be tangential or even irrelevant to the biography being told. Some element of selection is not only necessary but mandatory. A possible way out of this conundrum for the would-be biographer might be forthcoming from some recent developments in philosophy, specifically in the field of ontology.

In his book *Immaterialism*, the philosopher Graham Harman adopts a biological model to support his object-oriented ontology:

> If we treat every relation as significant for its *relata*, we slip into a "gradualist" ontology in which every moment is just as important as every other. ... A better model ... can be found in the Serial Endosymbiosis Theory ... the gradual shaping of the gene pool through natural selection is a less important evolutionary force than the watershed symbioses of distinct organisms. The idea has obvious value beyond the sphere of evolutionary biology: *in human biography, for instance* [my italics].[5]

Serial Endosymbiosis Theory (SET), initially developed by Lynn Sagan (later Lynn Margulis; 1938–2011), posited that the organelles of eukaryotic cells originated as independent creatures which then became subordinate components of the cell,[6] an idea now largely accepted in biology.

Adapting SET to his immaterialist theory, Harman envisages symbiosis as a special type of relation that changes the reality of one of its relata, change leading to an object/subject different in kind from what has gone before. Involving elements of chance, and generally occurring prior to maturity, symbiotic transformations are, in Harman's view, identifiable by their irreversibility, moving the object/subject to a new biographical stage, all impediments to final form removed. Harman suggested that perhaps two symbioses should be sought amongst each category of persons, places, and things[7] (hence possibly akin to Kipling's Who, Where, and What). He has given exemplars of this approach to history in accounts of the Dutch East India Company[8] and the American Civil War,[7] but his passing suggestion that symbioses might be relevant to human biography remains, to my knowledge, unexplored.

To illustrate the potentiality of this symbiotic approach to medical biography, a preliminary attempt at its application is suggested here, based on the life of Matthew Baillie (1761–1823), a notable physician of the late 18th and early 19th century,[9] whose career I have recently [2022] studied in collaboration with my colleague Professor Miratul Muqit,[10] and the 200th anniversary of whose death falls in 2023 (23rd September).

In Baillie's case, symbioses in the person category are obvious: he was the nephew of William Hunter (1718–1783) and John Hunter (1728–1793), two of the most notable names in 18th century medicine. Following the death of Baillie's father when he was 17, William Hunter paid for his nephew's education, facilitated his move from the University of Glasgow to a scholarship at Balliol College Oxford, encouraged him to study medicine, and in 1780 took him into his London home. In Baillie's autobiographical memoranda he states that Hunter was "the relation who had it most in his power to be useful to me with regard to my future prospects, … this determined me to enter the Medical Profession – I had no strong liking for this Profession … but I had no dislike to it, and I enter'd upon it willingly". Evidently then, this relationship was transformative. Likewise, John Hunter was able to facilitate his nephew's clinical training at St George's Hospital in London and subsequent appointment as physician there in 1787.

As for places which might be termed symbiotic in Baillie's biography, one can safely exclude the University of Oxford where Baillie considered that science was "very little cultivated" during his time there. A more promising candidate is William Hunter's Great Windmill Street Anatomy School. It was here, in the early 1780s, that Baillie first learned anatomy through dissection and, following in his uncle William's footsteps, became a noted teacher of the subject. In similar vein, his experience gained thereafter in the post-mortem room at St George's Hospital added to Baillie's knowledge: "I was not only as attentive as I could be to the Cases of my Patients, but embraced every opportunity of examining the Morbid appearances after death". These experiences culminated in his most significant contribution, *The Morbid Anatomy of some of the most important parts of the human body* (1793).[11] Considered to be one of the first comprehensive texts on the subject, it was supplemented with *A Series of Engravings Accompanied with Explanations which are Intended to Illustrate the Morbid Anatomy of some of the Most Important Parts of the Human Body*, published in fasciculi between 1799–1802.

As for the category of symbiotic things, the most obvious candidates are cadavers, either those obtained following the death of hospital patients as a consequence of disease or, probably more significantly, those obtained from resurrection men for the work of the Anatomy School. There is no doubt that Baillie, like his uncles, had dealings with such men in order to obtain sufficient material for dissection and study.

It may be disingenuous to suggest that an approach to medical biography seeking symbioses is novel, since this methodology is what many biographers already do in actuality in the analysis of their subject. Likewise, there may be other ways of conceptualising this approach, such as the framework of liminality analysis, wherein the idea of a threshold, inherent in the word liminal, indicates the possibility of change, transformation, or transition to a new state of being.[12]

Acknowledgement

Adapted and extended from: Larner AJ. Medical biography: a symbiotic methodology? *J Med Biogr* 2023;31:76–77.

References

1. Connor H. The *Journal of Medical Biography* is 30 years old: Past Achievements and Future Prospects. *J Med Biogr* 2023; **31**: 2–3.
2. Baron-Cohen S. *The pattern seekers. A new theory of human invention.* London: Penguin, 2022:14–15.
3. Seymour CA. *Introduction to clinical clerking.* Cambridge: Cambridge University Press, 1984.
4. Fisher CAH, Larner AJ. FAQs: memory loss. *Practitioner* 2006; **250**(1683): 14–16,19,21.
5. Harman G. *Immaterialism.* Cambridge: Polity Press, 2016:45–46.
6. Sagan L. On the origin of mitosing cells. *J Theoret Biol* 1967; **14**: 255–274.
7. Harman G. *Object-oriented ontology. A new theory of everything.* London: Pelican, 2018:114–134.
8. Harman G. *Immaterialism.* Cambridge: Polity Press, 2016:35–114.
9. Hill B. "Enlightened and honourable". Matthew Baillie, M.D. 1761–1823. *Practitioner* 1978; **220**: 490–493.

10. Muqit MMK, Larner AJ. Matthew Baillie (1761–1823): From Shotts to Duntisbourne Abbots. *Scott Med J* 2022; **67**: 129–133.

11. Hill, op. cit., ref. 9, p. 492, erroneously dates the publication of *Morbid Anatomy* as 1795.

12. Fisher HJ. Liminality, *hijra*, and the city. *Asian and African Studies* 1986; **20**: 153–177.

2. Liminality analysis: a conceptual framework applicable to medical biography?

> Always in life there are turning points, fateful beginnings which somehow seal your future – a moment that lets the future in, to paraphrase Grahame Greene.[1]

What is liminality? The word derives from limen, a Latin word meaning a threshold. Hence, in physiology a limen or liminal point is a sensory threshold of a physiological or psychological response; a stimulus may be described as infra-liminal if sub-threshold. Likewise, certain medical conditions, states, or contexts may be described as liminal, meaning on the threshold, at a boundary, on the margin, or transitional. For example, the syndrome of mild cognitive impairment has been described as a liminal state between full cognitive health and dementia.[2] Gibbons et al. have used the concept of liminality to explore the transition into a caregiving role experienced by informal caregivers.[3] In the context of medical history, Michel Foucault spoke of "la situation *liminaire* du fou a l'horizon du souci de l'homme médiéval",[4] which has been translated as "the *liminal* situation of the mad in medieval society" (Foucault's italics).[5]

Liminality analysis as a methodology originated in the domain of cultural anthropology, the key exponents in its development being Arnold van Gennep (1873–1957) and Victor W. Turner (1920–1983). Briefly stated, van Gennep (1909) characterised rites of passage as a transition through successive preliminal, liminal (or threshold), and postliminal stages, also designated separation, transition, and incorporation (or re-incorporation). The liminal period denoted a transition of undetermined duration from one state into another (e.g. adulthood, marriage), wherein an individual stands at a threshold with the prospect of something new, the crossing of which reconstructs their identity irreversibly.[5] Turner's work, examining ritual processes in tribal cultures, took van Gennep's triad as its starting point, characterising the liminal phase as a movement of separation from one structure to incorporation into another, distinct structure, during which individuals were "betwixt and between", not part of the society they previously belonged to yet not reincorporated into a new society.

It is now recognised that liminality analysis as a conceptual framework may be applied to an extraordinarily wide range of divergent situations including, as pointed out by Humphrey Fisher, both spatial and intellectual transitions.[7–9] It has, for example, been suggested, in passing, that it might be used in medical biography.[10] To illustrate the potentiality of liminality analysis in this context, a preliminary attempt at its application is made here by considering a period in the biography of the neurologist and physiologist David Ferrier (1843–1928).

Ferrier was eventually much celebrated (indeed knighted, 1911), his scientific reputation based on his experimental studies of localisation of motor and sensory functions in the brain, beginning in 1873 at the West Riding Asylum in Wakefield, West Yorkshire,[11] and his neurological reputation sealed by his appointment as a physician at the National Hospital, Queen Square, London, from 1880 to 1907. However, in the period between his qualification in medicine in Edinburgh in 1868 and his first appointment in London in 1870 as Lecturer in Physiology at the Middlesex Hospital, the direction of his career was uncertain.

A contemporary witness noted that after Ferrier's graduation with first class honours he was assistant to Thomas Laycock (1812–1876), Chair of the Practice of Physic at Edinburgh University from 1855, who had initiated instruction in medical psychology and mental diseases at Edinburgh. Ferrier's notes describing some of Laycock's treatments were used for publications in the *British Medical Journal* (1869;1:9 and 1869;2:8) but he undertook no original research at this time. Ferrier also "used to take the Friday afternoon lecture, and summarised Laycock's lectures for the previous week".[12] Apparently, however, "Wearied ... with the drudgery of tutorial work, which absorbed all his time",[13] Ferrier left Edinburgh in 1869. He then worked as an assistant to Dr William Edmund Image (1807–1903), a well-respected medical practitioner in Bury St. Edmunds in Suffolk, who was an acknowledged expert in forensic medicine and poisoning cases. (A later, secondary source says Ferrier took this post for financial reasons.[14]) Image later provided Ferrier with the post-mortem material which formed the basis for what may well be his first independent publication.[15]

That Ferrier found the work of general practice not entirely congenial is hinted at in some of his obituaries: he realised "that this was not his metier"[16] and "Image soon realized that Ferrier's abilities called for a wider scope, and he encouraged him to devote himself to research."[17] To this end, Ferrier spent much of his time writing his thesis, "largely amid the amenities of Image's garden" as he later recounted,[18] which was entitled "The comparative anatomy and intimate structure of the corpora quadrigemina" and won the Edinburgh gold medal in 1870. In the same year, Ferrier moved to London where he worked with the distinguished physician and experimentalist John Burdon Sanderson (1828–1905), and also encountered John Hughlings Jackson (1835–1911), already on the staff at Queen Square, who was to influence his views on neurology and his subsequent experimental work on the brain.[19] By 1871 Ferrier had been appointed to King's College London, where he stayed for the rest of his career, which was to include election to fellowships of the Royal Society (1876) and the Royal College of Physicians (1877), delivery of the Croonian Lecture at the Royal Society (1874, 1875), and of the Gulstonian (1878), Croonian (1890) and Lumleian (1906) Lectures at the Royal College of Physicians, as well as the Harveian Oration (1902), and the Presidency of the Neurological Society of London (1894) and of the Medical Society of London (1913–1914).

Applying liminality analysis, I suggest that Ferrier's time in Bury St Edmunds, far from being an inconsequential interlude (not even mentioned in his *BMJ* obituary: 1928;1:525–6), was in fact formative in the sense of being a liminal stage or situation between the preliminal and postliminal stages of, respectively, Edinburgh and London. Characteristic of a liminal stage, as defined by anthropologists and historians,[6,7] 1869–70 was an ambiguous period for Ferrier. The possibility of change, of entering or transitioning into a new state of being, lay before him, but his ultimate prospect was undefined, at least initially. In passing through this liminal phase, crossing this threshold, he committed to a career as an experimentalist and as a clinical neurologist; had he chosen general practice it is possible, even likely, that he would be all but unknown to posterity.

Perhaps it might be thought that, tentative though it is, this formulation stretches the horizons of liminality analysis too far. To my knowledge, there are no contemporaneous sources, either from Ferrier or others, describing his time in Bury St Edmunds, but that said it was evidently neither unstructured nor invisible, as per van Gennep's characterisation of the liminal phase, although clearly separated from his previous life and relatively secluded from centres of medical power and influence. Nevertheless, I suggest that the application of liminality analysis to medical biography may detect the presence of liminal periods, events, or situations in many careers.

How does liminality analysis compare with a previous proposal advocating a "symbiotic" approach[10] to biography? There are similarities, but also differences. As with symbiosis, liminality analysis can describe transitions which are subject to elements of chance, are irreversible, and move the subject to a new biographical stage. The symbiotic categories of places and things may correspond to liminal situations and events. However, symbiosis does not engage with the triad of stages of liminality analysis, stages which of themselves might be regarded as essential for an adequate contextualisation of any biographical transition.

Acknowledgements

I am indebted to the late Dr Humphrey Fisher (1933–2019) for introducing me to liminality many years ago (any errors in the foregoing analysis are strictly my own). Adapted and extended from: Larner AJ. Liminality analysis: a conceptual framework applicable to medical biography? *Journal of Medical Biography* 2024; **32**: 357–358.

References

1. Dafydd F. The girl who went into the East: a student's guide to R.S. In: Barnie J (ed). *Encounters with R.S. R.S. Thomas at 100.* Swansea: H'mm Foundation, 2013:36–42 [at 38]. The quotation from Greene's *The Power and the Glory* (1940) reads "There is always one moment in childhood when the door opens and lets the future in". Interestingly, Dafydd also uses the word "liminal" in her description [at 39] of arriving in Bangor on the very day that the death of R.S. Thomas was announced. In the same volume, Jon Gower describes the Llŷn peninsula as "a liminal place" [at 82].
2. Isaacs JD. Mild cognitive impairment: not much harm; not much help. *BJPsych Open* 2023; **9(6)**: e184.
3. Gibbons SW, Ross A, Bevans M. Liminality as a conceptual frame for understanding the family caregiving rite of passage: an integrative review. *Res Nurs Health* 2014; **37**: 423–436.
4. Scull A. *The insanity of place/The place of insanity. Essays on the history of psychiatry.* London: Routledge, 2006:37.
5. Foucault M. *History of madness.* London: Routledge, 1961 [2006]:11.
6. van Gennep A (transl. Vizedon MB, Caffee GL). *The rites of passage.* Chicago: University of Chicago Press, 1909 [1960].
7. Fisher HJ. Liminality, *hijra*, and the city. *Asian and African Studies* 1986; **20**: 153–177.
8. Fisher D. Liminality: the vocation of the Church (I). *Cistercian Studies Quarterly* 1989; **24**: 181–205.
9. Fisher D. Liminality: the vocation of the Church (II). The desert image in early medieval monasticism. *Cistercian Studies Quarterly* 1990; **25**: 188–218.
10. Larner AJ. Medical biography: a symbiotic methodology? *J Med Biogr* 2023; **31**: 76–77.
11. Larner AJ. A month in the country: the sesquicentenary of David Ferrier's classical cerebral localisation researches of 1873. *J R Coll Physicians Edinb* 2023; **53**: 128–131
12. Bramwell B. The Edinburgh Medical School and its professors in my student days (1865–1869). *Edinb Med J* 1923; **30**: 133–156.
13. Leyland J. (ed.). *Contemporary medical men and their professional work: biographies of leading physicians and surgeons, with portraits, from the*

"*Provincial Medical Journal*". *Volume II.* Leicester: Office of the Provincial Medical Journal, 1888: 61–67.

14. James FE. *The life and work of Thomas Laycock (1812–1876).* Unpublished PhD thesis, University of London, 1996. https://discovery.ucl.ac.uk/id/eprint/1318051/ [at 364].

15. Ferrier D. The trial for murder at Barsham. *Lancet* 1870; **2**: 350–351.

16. https://history.rcplondon.ac.uk/inspiring-physicians/sir-david-ferrier (accessed 05/12/23)

17. Stewart TG. Sir David Ferrier, LL.D., Sc.D., M.D., F.R.C.P., F.R.S. 1843–1928. *J Ment Sci* 1928; **74**: 375–380.

18. Sherrington CS. Sir David Ferrier, 1843–1928. *Proc R Soc Lond B Biol Sci* 1928; **103**: viii-xvi.

19. Ferrier D. Cerebral localisation in relation to therapeutics: being the Cameron Lecture of the University of Edinburgh, delivered February 26, 1892. *Edinb Med J* 1892; **37**: 881–897 [at 884].

3. Retrodiagnosis: the ontological, the epistemic, and the ethical

Abstract

Retrospective diagnosis of historical figures constitutes a well-developed historiography in the medical literature. However, these formulations are controversial, particularly to historians, on the grounds of unjustified assumption and anachronism. This communication explores potential ways to reconcile these positions, using the framework of ontological, epistemic and ethical considerations or challenges, first outlined by Muramoto, as sources of uncertainty. Of these, the ethical challenge should be addressed first, specifically to establish justifiable scholastic reasons for undertaking retrospective diagnosis. The ontological challenge may be addressed through a hybrid ontology which acknowledges both temporally-defined disease categories as artificial creations and the pre-existent natural facticity of disease entities which are relatively atemporal, allowing a possible escape from the charge of anachronism. The epistemic challenge depends upon the availability and interpretation of appropriate sources. A worked example illustrates how these challenges may be addressed in practice.

Introduction

Much of the business of clinical medicine consists of listening to a patient's account of their medical history (anamnesis) as a prelude to diagnosis, construction of a differential diagnosis, planning of investigations, and initiation of treatment. Although usually performed face-to-face, the COVID-19 pandemic has required us to become familiar with undertaking this process in spatially remote format (telephone, video link). Other narratives, temporally remote, may also be subjected to similar analysis, including biographical and autobiographical accounts, and historical documents, sometimes relating to individuals long dead, as well as fictional accounts which may have been based on experience rather than imagination. This may be described as retrospective diagnosis, also known as posthumous diagnosis or retrodiagnosis. We are deeply indebted to the work of Osamu Muramoto,[1] as acknowledged in my title and in the following exposition, for a carefully reasoned approach to this controversial topic.

Retrospective diagnoses are not hard to locate in the medical literature; they constitute a well-developed historiography. Speaking only of cognitive neurology, my own field of specialist interest, examples abound. To mention just a few: Jonathan Swift, author of *Gulliver's Travels*, has been retrospectively diagnosed as having frontotemporal dementia,[2] likewise the philosopher Friedrich Nietzsche, rather than neurosyphilis, as was previously widely thought.[3] Michael Faraday's mid-life loss of memory has been ascribed to a transient ischaemic attack in the vertebrobasilar arterial system.[4] Agatha Christie's celebrated disappearance for eleven days in December 1926 has been ascribed to functional (dissociative) amnesia.[5]

All these accounts of retrospective diagnosis were published in highly reputable, peer-reviewed journals by highly respected clinicians. So, may we reasonably conclude that retrospective diagnosis is, at worst, a harmless armchair pursuit, and at best a serious inquiry into the history of medicine? There are some strong objections, vigorously expressed. For example, Andrew Cunningham questioned whether retrospective diagnosis is legitimate, possible or desirable, opining that for historical purposes people die of what bystanders, medically qualified or not, say they died of, and hence as recorded in Bills of Mortality, Registrar-General reports, or statistics based on the International Classification of Diseases.[6] Evidently, then, Cunningham has not only no place for but also no concept of misdiagnosis or second opinions. Axel Karenberg considered retrospective diagnosis mere speculation, if sometimes erudite speculation, since the use of modern concepts of disease backwards in time represented "sources of unjustified assumption," presumably meaning anachronism. He went as far as to recommend that journal editors reject such papers when submitted.[7]

So, can these opposing positions be reconciled? Ian Hacking stated that "The impossibility of retroactive diagnosis is the academically correct, official history-of-medicine or philosophy-of-science teaching" but nevertheless opines that "we can say some things about old cases in the light of present experience".[8] One might also perhaps point out that all diagnosis is, to a certain extent, retrospective, looking back (anamnesis) on past events, as previously mentioned. But for a more carefully argued approach, we must engage with three particular challenges to retrospective diagnosis as identified by Osamu Muramoto: ontological; epistemic and ethical.[1] Although the first two of these, both sources of uncertainty, are my principal focus here, since making diagnostic judgments under uncertainty is familiar territory to practicing clinicians,[9] this is not to undervalue the ethical, as will become apparent in a brief worked example.

Ontological

Ontological (or aleatory, or first-order) uncertainty arises from the nature of reality; it is rooted in the basic structures of reality and is thus irreducible.[9] In the context of retrospective diagnosis, the ontological challenge asks whether disease entities persist over time.

Here is a celebrated example, from the French philosopher Bruno Latour's (1947–2022) paper "On the partial existence of existing and non-existing objects" in which he examined the case of Ramses (or Ramesses) II, a pharaoh of the nineteenth dynasty who ruled *ca.* 1279–1213 BCE. Following an examination of Ramses' mummy in 1976, the pharaoh was diagnosed as suffering from tuberculosis, prompting Latour to question "How could he [Ramses] have died of a bacillus discovered in 1882 [by Robert Koch] and of a disease whose etiology, in its modern form, dates only from 1819 in Laënnec's ward?"[10] Latour therefore contended that Ramses could not die of tuberculosis before its discovery: "Koch bacilli have a local history that limits them to Berlin at the turn of the century. They may be allowed to spread to all the years that come *after* 1882 … but … they cannot jump back to the years *before*." (italics in original).

Others share similar or overlapping views: for example, the historian Charles E. Rosenberg stated that "in some ways disease does not exist until we have agreed that it does, by perceiving, naming, and responding to it."[11] In similar vein, Annemarie Mol's fascinating study considers "atherosclerosis" as the correlate of particular diagnostic practices rather than as a disease-in-itself, enacted in different ways by different individuals; these alternative configurations indicate a multiple ontology.[12]

If accepted, arguments such as these would render attempts at retrospective diagnosis not merely problematic or misguided but entirely invalid. But counterarguments are available, for example from the philosopher Graham Harman:

> Atherosclerosis [*contra* Mol?] and tuberculosis [*contra* Latour?] are not produced *ex nihilo* in the medical practices that first register their existence; rather, these diseases as encountered in practice transform some genuine pre-existent entity or entities that our experience translates more or less capably. ... What we must not do is decapitate all talk of the disease in its own right, as if illness existed only as the retroactive sidekick of human medical officials. ... we should view it as ... strange to think that the disease itself is first born at the moment when humans detect it. Latour often ventures such claims ....[13]

Likewise, the historian David Wootton believes that "Latour's historicism misses a key point about science, which is that it is about matters which are the case whether we believe them to be so or not. ... he thinks discovery and invention are the same thing. They are not. ... science as a system of knowledge is more than a social construct because it is successful, because it fits with reality".[14]

Note that these arguments effectively distinguish between "disease categories" as human constructs which change across time and "disease entities" as pre-existent or evolving: the former are invented, the latter discovered. As clinicians we are of course aware that diseases may come and go (e.g. epidemics) even though there is probably little change in human biology over historical time and culture (i.e. it is transhistorical and transcultural), albeit some predispositions or vulnerabilities to disease, perhaps related to genetic make-up, may vary between times and places, related to evolutionary pressures or social conditions. Thus, Cunningham's argument that disease is not a-cultural or a-social[6] holds true for disease categories, but not for disease entities. I think this position is also consistent or congruent with the American philosopher Saul Kripke's (1940–2022) concept of "a posteriori necessity".[15] Our diagnoses are not known a priori, independent of experience. The necessary truth of a diagnosis is only revealed by empirical research, and the fact that we know anything is contingent – we might never have discovered it. Hence, the biography of a disease, like that of an historical figure, is contingent.

To reconcile these ontological stances, I suggest that recourse to a "hybrid ontology" may assist. In its original usage by Robert Brain, hybrid ontology was defined as a status which is "suspended between natural facticity and artificial creation".[16] In the context of diagnosis, appeal to a hybrid ontology would therefore characterize diagnosis as both natural facticity and artificial creation.

As such, one may argue that Ramses' diagnosis both is, and is not, tuberculosis. Ramses both has tuberculosis, considered as "natural facticity," a pre-existent disease entity; and does not have tuberculosis, considered as "artificial creation," a temporally-defined disease category.

These two (apparently) mutually contradictory states may immediately remind us of a famous thought experiment addressing just such a situation, viz. Schrödinger's Cat, conceptualizing the quantum mechanical phenomenon of superposition. Schrödinger's cat, placed in a closed box with a phial of poison which may break open at a random time, may be considered to be both alive and dead until the box is opened (i.e. a measurement is made). Diagnosis as hybrid ontology would permit the patient to both have and not have a particular diagnosis. Dependent upon the exact moment in history when clinicians open the diagnostic box, Ramses diagnosis either is (disease entity) or is not (disease category) tuberculosis, i.e. his diagnosis is both pre-existent (disease entity) and historically contingent (disease category). Hence, this formulation (which I tentatively label "Schrödinger's differential diagnosis" in contradistinction to differential diagnosis applying the law of parsimony, or Ockham's razor) argues for diseases as both pre-existent of their historical description, and capable of retroactive effects after their historical description, accepting that this relation is in tension with, but not invalidated by, arguments against anachronism. Diagnosis can then, in some manner, escape its temporal specificity.

Epistemic

Epistemic (or epistemological, or second-order) uncertainty arises from the nature of the evidence, the limitations in the current state of knowledge, arising from indeterminability or intractability.[9]

In the context of retrospective diagnosis, the epistemic challenge asks whether disease entities can be empirically verified retrospectively. If the ontological challenge has been successfully met, such that disease entities are acknowledged to have existed before their clinical description and incorporation into evolving nosologies, then the central challenge to retrospective diagnosis is epistemic.[17]

This might appear hopeless, since as we were not there, we cannot know: "any proposition about the past is formally unknowable, since we can't go back there to find out" as pointed out by a former President of the Classical Association, T.P. Wiseman. This claim, if valid, would render all historical study impossible, as irretrievable. However, as Wiseman continues, "meaningful statements about the past can be made, and constantly are made even by the most theoretical of us".[18]

In the context of retrospective diagnosis, the technological developments of modern biomedical science have enabled more precise diagnoses from the past to be discovered (NB not invented). To select just a few examples of paleopathology, which span the spectrum from disease pandemic to individual pathology: the origins of the Black Death in central Eurasia, based on genomic data from 14th century burials identifying *Y. pestis*;[19] the molecular identification of Paget's disease in the remains of medieval monks living at Norton Priory in Runcorn;[20] molecular genetic diagnosis of the scientist John Dalton's (1766–1844) colour blindness (daltonism),[21] or of Alois Alzheimer's first patient, Auguste D., whose archival brain tissue was found to show the typical features of Alzheimer's disease and to have a sequence variant, possibly a point mutation, in the presenilin-1 gene, one of the genes known to be deterministic for autosomal dominant Alzheimer's disease.[22] Ramses tuberculosis diagnosis 3000 years after his death might also be deemed to fall within this category, and thus to illustrate the linkage between the ontological and epistemic, in that resolution of epistemic uncertainty may also resolve ontological uncertainty.

Given the right conditions, DNA can last for centuries, even millennia. However, access to such material is not always available, and moreover not all conditions are susceptible to molecular (retro-)diagnosis. Many neurological and psychiatric syndromic diagnoses are entirely dependent upon history (anamnesis) alone. Hence it has been argued that retrospective syndromic diagnosis is feasible,[1] for example based on written accounts or, possibly, visual portrayals. This will, of course, as for molecular diagnosis, depend upon the available resources, which may change over time.

Ethical

The ethical challenge asks whether the lack of "patient" consent, the absence of a doctor-patient relationship, invalidates the whole process of retrospective diagnosis. For example, Simon Baron-Cohen has written that "diagnosis based on fragmentary biographical information is unreliable and arguably unethical, since diagnosis should always include the consent of the person and be initiated by them".[23] (But note the temporal specificity of this argument: within living memory, patients were routinely reported in the medical literature without application for consent either by the reporting clinician(s) or the publishing journal.) We are all familiar with the Goldwater Rule from the American Psychiatric Association's Principles of Medical Ethics which states, *inter alia*, that psychiatrists "should not give a professional opinion about public figures whom they have not examined in person, and from whom they have not obtained consent to discuss their mental health in public statements," a precept also supported by the Royal College of Psychiatrists. Similarly, the American Medical Association's Code of Medical Ethics (2017) states that physicians should refrain "from making clinical diagnoses about individuals (e.g. public officials, celebrities, persons in the news) they have not had the opportunity to personally examine".

Very occasionally an explicit statement to the effect that an individual wants their case history to be used for medical purposes may be available, e.g. the author Margiad Evans (1909–1958) specifically addressed *The Nightingale Silenced*, the second of her manuscripts describing her experience of epilepsy (following *A Ray of Darkness* in 1952), to medical professionals, motivated by "the desire to put into physicians' hands a book of clues to the sensations of such an epileptic as myself".[24] Dalton instructed that his eyes be examined after his death[21] (writing in 1873, the pathologist Thomas McDowall stated that "So far as is known, Dalton is the only colour-blind person who had a post-mortem examination performed for the express purpose of discovering the material cause of his defect of vision"[25]), although he cannot have imagined what investigations might have been available to posterity. But these cases of what might be termed proleptic consent or advance directive are exceptional. So how might we address the ethical challenge?

Muramoto argued that "there should be a justifiable scholastic reason that is carefully balanced against potential ethical concerns before initiating … medical evaluation in the absence of the patient's consent" and he presented possible purposes for making a retrospective diagnosis in a historical figure.[1] Issues to be taken into account include, but are not limited to, whether historical celebrities are immune to considerations of privacy (e.g. long dead, no risk of harm to the patient's reputation, or to living descendants) and/or has been subject to previous biography. Perhaps the 100–year embargo on public access to documents containing or suspected to contain personal information of people who may be living should be applied, *mutatis mutandi*, in cases of retrospective diagnosis.

Worked example: Faraday revisited

One of the examples of retrospective diagnosis mentioned previously was Michael Faraday's memory problems, specifically the clinical formulation made by the psychiatrist Edward Hare (1917–1996), first presented at the Royal Society of Medicine in 1974.[4] As these clinical symptoms fall within my area of specialist clinical interest, I have revisited this "case" and attempted a different formulation, to the effect that, rather than amnesia due to a transient ischaemic attack in the vertebrobasilar arterial system,[4] Faraday had a functional memory disorder.[26] This formulation was presented in light of

Muramoto's ontological, epistemic, and ethical challenges to retrospective diagnosis.

To take these in a different order, the ethical challenge is privileged here since there can be no doubt that this should (now) precede all other considerations. As a major figure in the history of chemistry and physics, Faraday may be deemed a legitimate subject of study, indeed has been the subject of many biographies, some of which have specifically addressed his health issues. It is over 150 years since his death (1867) and he had no children so has no direct descendants. From the broader scholarly view, as advocated by Muramoto,[1] retrospective diagnosis might help us to understand the influence of illness on his work (or lack of it for a period of around 2 years).

As regards the ontological challenge, the question is whether or not functional cognitive disorders existed in the 19th century. Whilst the categorization is relatively new (2015),[27] there seems little reason to doubt that such symptoms have always been part of the human condition (and ever will be).

As regards the epistemic challenge, the question is whether or not there is sufficient evidence to sustain the syndromic diagnosis on a probabilistic (Bayesian) basis (unlike the apodistic, categorical, true/false diagnosis which may be possible with molecular retrodiagnoses). This is dependent on the available documentary evidence surviving in the historical record, from Faraday himself and collateral sources (and the diligence, or otherwise, of the researcher in tracking down this evidence). Of note in this context, Muramoto has opined that syndromic diagnosis of functional disorders is "a highly useful construction of the state of affairs of the patient" and can be made from history alone[1] (as seen with the retrospective diagnosis of functional amnesia in Agatha Christie[5]). Ultimately of course, it is for the reader to determine whether this diagnostic formulation is deemed more likely to be discovery (natural facticity) or invention (artificial creation).

Conclusion

Retrospective diagnosis is a contested field, with different perspectives amongst medical historians and clinicians (lay historians). The discussion presented here argues that there are legitimate circumstances for attempting retrospective diagnosis, taking into account ethical, ontological, and epistemic challenges.

Acknowledgement

This is the substance (not transcript) of a lecture delivered at a webinar of the History of Medicine Society, Royal Society of Medicine, London, 15th March 2023. Unpublished.

References

1. Muramoto O. Retrospective diagnosis of a famous historical figure: ontological, epistemic, and ethical considerations. *Philos Ethics Humanit Med* 2014; 9: 10
2. Lorch M. Language and memory disorder in the case of Jonathan Swift: considerations on retrospective diagnosis. *Brain* 2006; 129: 3127–3137.
3. Orth M, Trimble MR. Friedrich Nietzsche's mental illness – general paralysis of the insane vs. frontotemporal dementia. *Acta Psychiatr Scand* 2006; 114: 439–444.
4. Hare EH. Michael Faraday's loss of memory. *Proc R Soc Med* 1974; 67: 617–618.
5. De Vito S, Della Sala S. Was Agatha Christie's mysterious amnesia real or revenge on her cheating spouse? *Scientific American Mind* 2017; 28(6): 30–34. https://www.scientificamerican.com/article/was-agatha-christie-rsquo-s-mysterious-amnesia-real-or-revenge-on-her-cheating-spouse/
6. Cunningham A. Identifying disease in the past: cutting the Gordian knot. *Asclepio* 2002; 54: 13–34.
7. Karenberg A. Retrospective diagnosis: use and abuse in medical historiography. *Prague Med Rep* 2009; 110: 140–145.
8. Hacking I. *Mad travellers. Reflections on the reality of transient mental illnesses*. London: Free Association Books, 1998: 87.
9. Han PKJ. *Uncertainty in medicine. A framework for tolerance*. Oxford: Oxford University Press, 2021.
10. Latour B. On the partial existence of existing and non-existing objects. In: Daston LJ (ed). *Biographies of scientific objects*. Chicago: University of Chicago Press, 2000: 247–269.
11. Rosenberg CE. Framing disease: illness, society and history. In Rosenberg CE, Golden JL (eds). *Framing disease: studies in cultural history*. New Brunswick, NJ: Rutgers University Press, 1992: xiii.
12. Mol A. *The body multiple: ontology in medical practice*. Durham, NC, and London: Duke University Press, 2002.
13. Harman G. *Immaterialism*. Cambridge: Polity Press, 2016: 43–44.
14. Wootton D. *The invention of science. A new history of the scientific revolution*. London: Penguin, 2016: 540.
15. Kripke SA. *Naming and necessity*. Cambridge: Harvard University Press, 1980.
16. Brain R. *The pulse of modernism: physiological aesthetics in fin-de-siecle Europe*. Seattle: University of Washington Press, 2015: xviii.
17. Larner AJ. Editorial: Retrospective diagnosis: pitfalls and purposes. *J Med Biogr* 2019; 27: 127–128.
18. Sommerstein AH. *Aristophanes. Lysistrata and other plays. The Acharnians, The Clouds, Lysistrata* (Revised edition). London, Penguin Books, 2002: xli (n22).
19. Spyrou MA, Musralina L, Gnecchi Ruscone GA, Kocher A, Borbone P-G,

Khartanovich VI, et al. The source of the Black Death in fourteenth-century central Eurasia. *Nature* 2022; 606: 718–724.

20. Shaw B, Burrell CL, Green D, Navarro-Martinez A, Scott D, Daroszewska A, et al. Molecular insights into an ancient form of Paget's disease of bone. *Proc Natl Acad Sci USA* 2019; 116: 10463–10472.

21. Hunt DM, Dulai KS, Bowmaker JK, Mollon JD. The chemistry of John Dalton's color blindness. *Science* 1995; 267: 984–988.

22. Müller U, Winter P, Graeber MB. A presenilin 1 mutation in the first case of Alzheimer's disease. *Lancet Neurol* 2013; 13: 129–130.

23. Baron-Cohen S. *The pattern seekers. A new theory of human invention.* London: Penguin, 2022: 80.

24. Pratt J (ed). *The Nightingale Silenced and other late unpublished writings by Margiad Evans.* Aberystwyth: Honno, 2020: 132.

25. McDowall TW. On the power of perceiving colours possessed by the insane. *West Riding Lunatic Asylum Medical Reports* 1873; 3: 129–152 [at 147].

26. Larner AJ. Michael Faraday's "loss of memory" revisited. *J Hist Neurosci* 2021; 30: 155–162.

27. Stone J, Pal S, Blackburn D, Reuber M, Thekkumpurath P, Carson A. Functional (psychogenic) cognitive disorders: a perspective from the neurology clinic. *J Alzheimers Dis* 2015; 48(Suppl1): S5–S17.

Coda

One vision of historical scholarship (e.g. E.H. Carr) is the combination of facts with interpretations. Medical historians originating in the medical tradition are sometimes accused of prioritising facts over interpretations (certainly I am guilty of this) whereas medical historians from the historical/humanities tradition may be more inclined to offer interpretations. Whichever, retrodiagnosis might be characterised as an attempt at interpretation in light of the factual evidence, rather than a hunt for the present in an earlier age (Butterworth).

4. Writing case reports: suggested methodology

Abstract

This communication briefly looks at the reasons for, and mechanics of, writing case reports and case series for publication. The author argues that this genre may be characterised as a stylised form of medical biography. As a narrative form of medical knowledge, case reporting is of value in the development of clinical reasoning skills.

Why report cases?

Before the "how to do it", it is necessary to ask the question: why do it? Case reports and case series constitute the lowest rung in the hierarchy of clinical evidence, for which reason they are derided in some quarters as mere anecdote. Indeed, some journals in which they were once a staple have abandoned publishing them altogether (on the other hand, some online journals devoted exclusively to the publication of case reports have started up in recent years). So, are there any valid reasons why we should continue to write case reports? The answer given here is an emphatic yes (perhaps to be anticipated, since the author has published at least one case report every year since 1988). This affirmation is based on a number of arguments,[1-3] not merely that this is a "rite of passage" for junior doctors wishing to ascend the clinical hierarchy:

- Awareness raising: a well-presented and plausibly argued case report can highlight specific learning points in diagnosis, investigation and management, and hence fulfil an important role in medical education, fostering the skills of clinical judgement.
- Cognitive purpose: very occasionally case reports present a hitherto undescribed entity and so advance medical knowledge: the written history of Parkinson's disease started with a series of six cases, three observed only in passing, using a so-called "street watch methodology";[4] the written history of Alzheimer's disease began with the clinico-pathological report of a single case.[5]
- Case reports may be used as arguments for proof of concept or, more plausibly based on the philosophical perspective of Karl Popper (1902–1994), refutation of concept. Exceptions to the expected may challenge widely accepted clinical diagnostic criteria.[6,7]
- Case reports may (as even proponents of evidence-based medicine acknowledge) act as hypothesis generators, a preliminary datum identifying problems to which research methodology can be subsequently applied. Case reports of suspected adverse drug reactions can be an important signal to prompt more systematic studies.[8]
- Narrative of individual cases ("Doctors' stories") is the idiom of clinical practice: it is what we attend to every working day.[9]

In addition to these arguments, it may also be worth considering case reports from the perspective of medical history: case reports and series may be seen as descendants emanating from the tradition of the *consilia* of the physicians of past centuries, in that both are examples of written texts responding to the particular case, offering practical clinical advice based on experiential observations.

In this communication some heuristic suggestions are proffered on how to go about preparing a case report or case series for publication (with the important proviso that these suggestions are not claimed in any way to guarantee success!), since this is a topic which does not generally feature in medical curricula. Some illustrations from the author's particular sphere of interest, neurology, are given, although similar arguments can assuredly be made for other clinical disciplines.

How to report cases?

Case selection is crucial: the key point is to identify the message you wish to convey, preferably before any writing up occurs. To borrow from Marshall McLuhan (1911–1980), when it comes to case reports the medium is the message, as exemplified in "Lesson of the Week/Month" columns which appear or have appeared in some journals.

If possible, identify your target journal early on (senior clinicians with experience of publication may be helpful in providing advice on this point) and adhere to its guidelines for authors with respect to word count, figures, references. Editors may be irritated by failure to comply with these guidelines and increasingly papers may be returned to authors without being sent for peer review if they are not adhered to. Most journals now require signed patient consent forms at initial manuscript submission, not after acceptance, so it is best to acquire these early on, before the patient is lost to follow up. Some journals, especially online productions, require a fee, often several hundred euros/dollars, for handling and publishing open access papers, so be aware of this and identify a reliable source of funding before you submit.

What cases to report?

Whilst highly unusual cases (so-called "fascinomas") may merit publication, they may be of limited heuristic value since the lessons to be drawn from them may not be easily generalised. Probably of more value, and hence greater chance of acceptance for publication, are cases detailing unusual features in common diseases[10] since awareness of the possible presentation of the underlying condition may thereby be increased. Such variant cases may be classified under the rubric of "broadening the phenotype".[11,12]

Reports which illuminate differential diagnosis have obvious teaching relevance,[13] and cases with initial diagnostic mistakes ("mea culpa") or misapprehensions can be particularly instructive, as well as chastening.[14] Illustrations of the clinical-anatomical methodology are much loved by neurologists, often now in the form of clinico-radiological correlations,[15–17] as opposed to clinico-pathological studies which often take much longer to reach diagnostic fruition.[6,18] Cases which reflect advances in the understanding of specific disorders, sometimes resulting in the deployment of new treatments,[19] are also potential fodder, as are therapeutic dilemmas which may illustrate deficiencies in the existing evidence base.[20] Prolonged follow-up of cases, ideally for decades,[21,22] may also be a productive field, particularly if the patient has previously been reported in the literature.[23-25]

Structuring the case report

Most case reports by convention follow a fairly standardised structure, a fixed regularity which befits this narrative genre,[9] each element of which is considered here in turn.

Title: This requires some careful thought. As we live in an "attention economy", with many demands upon these limited resources, the title may be all that the potential reader initially encounters. Accordingly, if you wish to be read, a short, pithy,[26] catchy (alliterative?), intriguing title[27] which summarises the report or its message,[28] even to the point of acting as an adage, may be deemed highly desirable, whereas "A case of such-and such a disease" may act as a turn off, giving the diagnostic game away at the outset. Interrogatives may also pique a reader's curiosity to pursue matters further.[18,26,29,30]

Abstract: Some, but not all, journals require an abstract for case reports, not least for indexing purposes. However, this does tell, albeit in abbreviated form, the story and removes all possibility of the suspense which an unabstracted case report can build in its movement toward the diagnostic denouement.

Introduction: This presents the background, setting the scene by relating what is already known, or in other words contextualising the case. This should be brief: an exhaustive literature review is not required. The reader should be left wanting more. It is desirable to conclude this section by briefly stating the aim(s) or objective(s) of the report.

Case Report(s): This is the meat of the piece, presenting the (anonymised) history, examination, and investigation findings, or in other words the clinical narrative. Since case data may have been gathered in a rather piecemeal, haphazard, way, depending on how the clinical scenario played out (and of course unlike the systematic data collection of clinical trials), it may appear difficult to tell a clearly evolving and coherent story. This is where the art of case reporting becomes most apparent: this is, after all, a construct which attempts an interpretive reconstruction of the actual case. There should be a rigorous pruning of all extraneous material, aside from a few judicious negatives. Specific dates should be avoided, it is better to give times from the onset of symptoms (e.g. "three months later"), in other words information should be presented chronologically. Failure to observe internal consistency in the case reportage will invite rejection.

Discussion: This should briefly summarize the particular case presented, and then contextualise it in the light of other similar cases, and state clearly the "take home" lesson(s) or message(s) to be learned from this case, perhaps in the form of recommendations for practice.

References: The citations will generally be focused rather than exhaustive, since there are often strictures on the number of references which may be cited. Note the particular reference style of your chosen journal and adhere to it.

Pragmatic considerations

Although writing up a case report or series may seem a straightforward proposition at the outset, this is not necessarily true. On occasion the pathway from idea to published article is smooth and brief (months), but often the road is bumpy and publication may easily take a year or more. Some journals have long delays even between acceptance and publication (my record is approaching 2 years, and counting), although articles may be available sooner on-line. Case reporting is not necessarily a speedy route to augmentation of your CV!

Even if the case notes are to hand, and the message to be conveyed is obvious from the outset, beginning the writing process, the challenge of the blank page, can be daunting for some would-be authors, however fluent they may be with the spoken word. Clarity of written presentation may not be immediately forthcoming, and more than one draft of the manuscript may be required prior to submission.

Dependent upon the complexity of the case and the involvement of other clinicians, the number of co-authors may expand, all of whom will need to make some contribution to and read the final manuscript, a factor which may slow progress: as the number of co-authors increases as an arithmetic progression, the time taken to finalise the submission may seem to increase as a geometric progression (I have experience of a senior co-author taking more than a year to getting around to reading a manuscript, and then having essentially nothing to contribute to it). Would-be "authors" may unexpectedly emerge from the woodwork as it becomes apparent that publication is a possibility, not having been previously apparent to do any of the work, at which point it may be sensible to consult the criteria for authorship enunciated by the International Committee of Medical Journal Editors, in short:

- Substantial contributions to the conception or design, or acquisition, analysis or interpretation of data;
- Drafting or revising the work for important intellectual content;
- Final approval of the version to be published;
- Agreement to be accountable for all aspects of the work.

Once submitted, rejection of the manuscript is a possibility to be anticipated, an event which, however initially galling, should, as for other life experiences, be handled philosophically (there is more than one journal in the world which may be interested to publish your work, and sometimes papers end up in better journals having been rejected elsewhere). Although reviewer comments often appear crass or wilfully obtuse, suggesting they have either not read or not understood the manuscript, there may sometimes be a useful suggestion which might facilitate later acceptance and should therefore be adopted if possible.

Resilience, a determination to battle on, sometimes amounting to bloody-mindedness, is sometimes required. If you have invested effort to write something up, then abandoning it might represent a waste of time, although most experienced authors will have consigned at least one proposed case report to the dustbin of history because of its unsuitability for publication (hence the critical importance of case selection mentioned previously). Acceptance is, of course, a joy (albeit often transient) and seeing ones name in print may give the impression that you are making some (minuscule) contribution to medical knowledge.

Discussion

The epistemological importance of narrative in clinical medicine is undisputed, hence the importance of case reports as a pedagogical and heuristic device.[9] Lest anyone should be too dismissive of this link between literature (rather than science) and medicine, it is well-recognised that the narrative description of disease in individual patients (the medical case) evolved at about the same time in the nineteenth century as detective fiction, both examples of case-based inquiry.[9,31] It is no coincidence that the methodology of Sherlock Holmes – a literary character created by a clinician, Arthur Conan Doyle (1859–1930), and based on his experience of Dr Joseph Bell (1837–1911), an Edinburgh physician[32] – namely, "the retrospective construction of a hypothetical narrative in order to work out the relation of the clues to one another within an acceptable chronology",[9] remains applicable in clinical practice and in the formulation of case reports. As Søren Kierkegaard (1813–1855) famously pointed out, "Life can only be understood backwards; but it must be lived forwards", a dictum which may underpin Holmes' reasoning backwards from effect to cause. The case report exemplifies this in many ways: the clinical scenario which may initially have baffled the clinician is retrospectively reported as a seemingly linear progression to diagnosis. The medical interpretation of the patient history creates a metastory of illness which facilitates understanding and, hopefully, treatment.

For these reasons, far from belittling the writing of case reports, this is a skill which should be encouraged in all clinicians.[33]

Acknowledgement

Adapted and extended from: Ghadiri-Sani M, Larner AJ. How to write a case report. *Br J Hosp Med* 2014;75:207–10.

References

1. Simpson RJ Jr, Griggs TR. Case reports and medical progress. *Perspect Biol Med* 1985; **28**: 402–6.
2. Vandenbroucke JP. In defense of case reports and case series. *Ann Intern Med* 2001; **134**: 330–4.
3. Miller R, Linssen R. The value of case reports in medical education. *Br J Hosp Med* 2013; **74**: 666.
4. Parkinson J. *An Essay on the Shaking Palsy 1817*. Chichester: Wiley-Blackwell, 2010.
5. Alzheimer A. Über eine eigenartige Erkrankung der Hirnrinde. *Allgemeine Zeitschrift fur Psychiatrie und Psychisch-Gerichtlich Medizine* 1907; **64**: 146–8.
6. Ali R, Barborie A, Larner AJ, White RP. Psychiatric presentation of sporadic Creutzfeldt-Jakob disease: a challenge to current diagnostic criteria. *J Neuropsychiatry Clinical Neurosci* 2013; **25**: 335–8
7. Larner AJ. Diagnostic criteria for sporadic Creutzfeldt-Jakob disease still missing psychiatric features. *Prog Neurol Psychiatry* 2022; **26**(3): 36.
8. Eke T, Talbot JF, Lawden MC. Severe persistent visual field constriction associated with vigabatrin. *BMJ* 1997; **314**: 180–1.
9. Hunter KM. *Doctors' stories. The narrative structure of medical knowledge*. Princeton: Princeton University Press, 1991.
10. Ramtahal J, Larner AJ. Diagnosing multiple sclerosis: expect the unexpected. *Br J Hosp Med* 2008; **69**: 230.
11. Doran M, Enevoldson TP, Ghadiali EJ, Larner AJ. Mills syndrome with dementia: broadening the phenotype of FTD/MND. *J Neurol* 2005; **252**: 846–7.

12. Ghadiri-Sani M, Waqar M, Smith D, Doran M. Paraneoplastic neurological syndromes: severe neurological symptoms resulting from relatively benign or occult tumours – two case reports. *Case Rep Oncol Med* 2013; **2013**: 458378.

13. Smithson E, Larner AJ. Glioblastoma multiforme masquerading as herpes simplex encephalitis. *Br J Hosp Med* 2013; **74**: 52–3.

14. Larner AJ. Getting it wrong: the clinical misdiagnosis of Alzheimer's disease. *Int J Clin Pract* 2004; **58**: 1092–4.

15. Larner AJ, Zeman AZJ, Antoun NM, Allen CMC. MRI appearances in subacute combined degeneration of the spinal cord due to vitamin B_{12} deficiency. *J Neurol Neurosurg Psychiatry* 1997; **62**: 99–100.

16. Ghadiri-Sani M, Dougan C, Lecky B. Slowly progressive upper limb weakness: two cases of Hirayama disease and review of literature. *J Neurol Neurosurg Psychiatry* 2013; **84**: e2

17. Larner AJ. Cerebral mass lesions presenting in a cognitive disorders clinic. *Br J Hosp Med* 2013; **74**: 694–5.

18. Menon R, Baborie A, Jaros E, Mann DMA, Ray PS, Larner AJ. What's in a name? Neuronal intermediate filament inclusion disease (NIFID), frontotemporal lobar degeneration-intermediate filament (FTLD-IF) or frontotemporal lobar degeneration-fused in sarcoma (FTLD-FUS)? *J Neurol Neurosurg Psychiatry* 2011; **82**: 1412–4.

19. Sells RAD, Larner AJ. From symptoms to causes: progress in the treatment of neurological disease. *Br J Hosp Med* 2011; **72**: 350–1.

20. Larner AJ, Rose EL, Humphrey PRD. A therapeutic dilemma: atrial fibrillation, transient ischaemic attacks, and an unruptured intracranial aneurysm. *Hosp Med* 2003; **64**: 52–3.

21. Larner AJ, Jacob A. Paroxysmal exercise-induced dystonia with optic atrophy: 30–year follow-up. *Neurol India* 2010; **58**: 135–6.

22. Aji BM, Ghadiali EJ, Jacob A, Larner AJ. Passage of an iron bar through the head: 50–year follow-up. *J Neurol* 2012; **259**: 1247–8.

23. Larner AJ, Moss J, Rossi ML, Anderson M. Congenital insensitivity to pain: a 20 year follow up. *J Neurol Neurosurg Psychiatry* 1994; **57**: 973–4.

24. Rawle MJ, Larner AJ. NARP syndrome: a 20–year follow-up. *Case Rep Neurol* 2013; **5**: 204–7.

25. Aung PP, Hamid S, Larner AJ. Later life cognitive impairment: an ophthalmological diagnostic clue? *Prog Neurol Psychiatry* 2019; **23**(4): 13–4.

26. Ramtahal J, Larner AJ. Shaky legs? Think POT! *Age Ageing* 2009; **38**: 352–3.

27. Larner AJ. Amnesia as a sex-related adverse event. *Br J Hosp Med* 2011; **72**: 292–3.

28. Larner AJ. Pitfalls in the diagnosis of ulnar neuropathy: remember the deep palmar branch. *Br J Hosp Med* 2010; **71**: 654–5.

29. Larner AJ, Thomas DJ. Can myasthenia gravis be diagnosed with the "ice pack test"? A cautionary note. *Postgrad Med J* 2000; **76**: 162–3.

30. Larner AJ. Braille alexia: an apperceptive tactile agnosia? *J Neurol Neurosurg Psychiatry* 2007; **78**: 907–8.

31. Kempster PA, Lees AJ. Neurology and detective writing. *Pract Neurol* 2013; **13**: 372–6.
32. Larner AJ. "Neurological literature": Sherlock Holmes and neurology. *Adv Clin Neurosci Rehabil* 2011; **11**(1): 20,22.
33. Anwar R, Kabir H, Botchu R, Khan SA, Gogi N. How to write a case report. *BMJ* 2003; **327**(suppl): s153–4.

Key points:

- Though dismissed by some as anecdote, case reports in fact reflect the idiom of clinical medicine: focusing the clinical gaze on the individual patient.
- Although not all cases are worthy of being written up, there are a number of reasons for seeking case publication, not least as a teaching resource.
- Case selection is critical: seek advice from a senior clinician with experience of the process on matters of the key message and suitable journal.
- Once a target journal is identified, following the rubric to the letter.
- If rejected, be persistent: if the case and its message is good enough, it will get published!

---

5. Prosopography versus biography in the history of neurology: a clinician's viewpoint

What is prosopography? Clinicians may be familiar with the "prosopo-" prefix, from conditions such as prosopagnosia, an inability to recognise faces which may be developmental or acquired in origin; and prosopoplegia, a facial weakness or paralysis, of which one cause is Bell's palsy.[1] Literally, then, prosopography would seem to imply "writing the face, or person", as per Quintilian's use of *prosopopeia* as a device in classical rhetoric dating from the first century CE.

Prosopography may be defined as a "description of a person's social and family connections, career, etc., or a collection of such descriptions". Thus defined, prosopography would seem to overlap, at least in part, with the processes of biography. However, the emphasis of prosopography is more on collective biography, rather than on a single individual. As such, the art or genre of prosopography has a long history, perhaps dating back to Plutarch's *Parallel Lives* from the first century CE. Giorgio Vasari's *Lives of the most excellent painters, sculptors, and architects* from the sixteenth century CE may also be deemed an example of prosopography. Another prominent example sometimes cited is Lewis Namier's work on members of the British House of Commons in the late 18th century. In the world of science, Robert K. Merton's early work on 17th century English Puritans who pursued scientific interests[2] is also within the prosopographical tradition.

What is the value of prosopography, as opposed to biography? In focussing on a single individual, biography may run the risk of decontextualising the subject, particularly if documenting a great man (*sic*) and his great deeds – the Whiggish approach. A particular risk here for clinicians with an interest in the history of medicine (as opposed to historians with an interest in the history of medicine) is that of self-identification with the biographical subject, a "faculty of self-projection, of discovering his own features in those of his subject" and hence of writing a "concealed autobiography".[3] In contrast, prosopography is focused on shared context, attempting to uncover common characteristics, patterns and relationships. As such it is applicable not only to powerful elites and the famous but also to "ordinary people", hence to social and economic rather than political history, as exemplified by the Annales school and the work of Emmanuel Le Roy Ladurie (1929–2023), *Montaillou, village occitan de 1294 à 1324* (published in 1975). Interest in the possibilities of extended prosopography, including in the domain of the history of science, has burgeoned in the past 50 years or so, stimulated by the work of a number of historians.[4-6]

Prosopography may appear in different forms, dependent upon parameters such as the aims of the historian and the data available. Indeed, a historiographic spectrum may be envisaged. At one end of this spectrum, the analysis may involve large numbers of individuals who have left little if any personal footprint in the historical record, other than perhaps administrative data. Here no biography may be required, necessary, or even possible. Analysis may be processual, possibly even automated and/or digital. At the other end of the spectrum, data available in the historical record for small groups, defined perhaps by profession or location, may permit some individual biography to be merged into the prosopographical process. Hence the notion of "collective biography" may be feasible, and medical history may be one sphere in which this might be of interest.

Whilst caution is obviously necessary when advocating any admixture of history and science, since previous opinions have differed markedly on the question of history as science,[7,8] nevertheless I venture to suggest a formulation of prosopography versus biography as different forms of historiography which is based on the medical model of clinical evidence.

Thus, individual biography may be conceptualized as akin to the presentation of a single case report or case study: this is instructive about the individual but does not necessarily provide any generalisable lesson(s), as implied in the terminology of "fascinoma" which is sometimes used of such medical cases (see also "Writing case reports: suggested methodology").[9]

In contrast, prosopography as a form of collective biography may be conceptualized as akin to clinical studies involving multiple individuals, ranging from the case series (anything from three to a few hundred) to the population-based study (involving thousands to hundreds of thousands). The latter may adopt a methodology in which data are anonymised, as for example in diagnostic or screening test accuracy studies, or randomised or open label therapeutic trials, or analysis of administrative healthcare data. This approach entails an increasing degree of generalisability or transfer of any outcome(s), but without necessarily being relevant or applicable to the individual case, since it is in the nature of generalisations always to have exceptions.

Accordingly, with these caveats, there is rationale for both approaches. Whereas a hierarchy of clinical evidence has been defined, wherein outcomes of larger studies have more significance and take precedence for deciding clinical actions or interventions in situations of uncertainty, no such hierarchy is necessary for biography and prosopography since these approaches are complementary, accepting that the breadth of the prosopographic approach may necessarily sacrifice some of the depth achievable in an individual biography.

As pointed out by Felix Goodbody, "prosopography is suited to the study of local medical networks".[10] It provides an opportunity to examine, where known, the social origins, training, and subsequent career trajectories of individuals in this specific employment group, searching for any commonalities as well as differences. As such, it is an eminently suitable methodology for an extended analysis of individuals working in a specific location and/or over a restricted time period. In my own studies, this comprises the clinicians both resident and either visiting or contributing to the work undertaken at the West Riding Lunatic Asylum at Wakefield in West Yorkshire between 1866 and 1876, encompassing the superintendency of James Crichton-Browne. According to E.D. Adrian, this was "the period when neurology became a science".[11] Whilst significant names in the history of neurology, such as John Hughlings Jackson and David Ferrier, were associated with the Asylum at this time, and contributed to its house journal, the *West Riding Lunatic Asylum Medical Reports*,[12] many other clinicians also worked there during this period. An extended prosopography, developed around individual biographies, may be of interest in understanding the development not only of this particular "research laboratory"[13] or "research school"[14] but also of neurology as an independent clinical discipline.

Acknowledgement

Unpublished manuscript, late-2023.

References

1. Larner AJ. *A dictionary of neurological signs* (4th edition). London: Springer, 2016: 261–262.
2. Merton RK. Science, technology and society in seventeenth-century England. *Osiris* 1938; 4: 360–632.
3. Nuttall AD. *Dead from the waist down. Scholars and scholarship in literature and the popular imagination.* New Haven and London: Yale University Press, 2003: 107, 146.
4. Stone L. Prosopography. *Daedalus* 1971; 100: 45–73.
5. Shapin S, Thackray A. Prosopography as a research tool in history of science: the British scientific community 1700–1900. *History of Science* 1974; 12: 1–28.
6. Pyenson L. "Who the guys were": prosopography in the history of science. *History of Science* 1977; 15: 155–188
7. Trevelyan GM. History and the reader. In: *An autobiography and other essays.* London: Longmans, Green and Co, 1949: 52–67 [esp. 52–57].
8. Greenaway F. The history of science and the science of history. *Proc R Inst GB* 1973; 46: 99–115.
9. Ghadiri-Sani M, Larner AJ. How to write a case report. *Br J Hosp Med* 2014; 75: 207–210.
10. Goodbody F. *Liverpool's medical community 1930–1998: social, knowledge and business networks.* Unpublished PhD thesis, University of Liverpool, 2020. https://livrepository.ac.uk/3093988/1/200871054_Jun2020.pdf [at 36].
11. Adrian ED. Ferrier Lecture. The localization of activity in the brain. *Proc R Soc Lond B Biol Sci* 1939; 126: 433–449 [at 433].
12. Larner AJ. The *West Riding Lunatic Asylum Medical Reports*: the precursor of *Brain*? *Brain* 2023; 146: 4437–4445.
13. Easterbrook CC. Sir James Crichton-Browne. *Edinb Med J* 1938; 45: 294–301 [at 297].
14. Finn MA. *The West Riding Lunatic Asylum and the making of the modern brain sciences in the nineteenth century.* Unpublished PhD thesis, University of Leeds, 2012. https://etheses.whiterose.ac.uk/3412/.

Robert Wilfred Skeffington Lutwidge (1802–1873)

When first encountered, this marvellous name will surely prompt the interest of anyone familiar with the name of the author Lewis Carroll, specifically his real name, as opposed to his pseudonym: Charles Lutwidge Dodgson. As Lutwidge is an unusual name, the possibility of a link is immediately suggested. Brief research will confirm a family relationship: R.W.S. Lutwidge was the uncle of Charles Dodgson ("uncle Skeffington"), his sister having married a Dodgson. But the family relationship is not the only reason that Lutwidge may be known to posterity.

He was a barrister by training, in which capacity he became involved with the workings of the Lunacy Acts, as a legal member of the Lunacy Commission, specifically Inquiry Commissioner in 1842, Secretary in 1845 to 1855, and thereafter Commissioner in Lunacy.[1] Some insights into his work in the capacity of Commissioner may be gained from the records of the asylums he visited. For example, he made the final visit, with Samuel Gaskell, to the Bedford Asylum on 22nd December 1859, prior to its closure in 1860 with removal of the patients to the new Three Counties Asylum in Arlesey.[2] (Peculiarly, in his history of Bedford Asylum, Cashman gives the name as "Lutteridge" and elsewhere as "W.S. Lutwidge".[3]) His report on the West Riding Asylum in Wakefield, which he visited from 9–11th March 1870, bore testimony to the "very creditable state of the Asylum".[4] A further positive report was issued following his visit of 10–11th November 1871.[5] Scrimgeour also gives an (earlier) example of Lutwidge's intervention to have a patient transferred from a local workhouse to Wakefield Asylum in 1858, even though the patient was not insane and was shortly thereafter freed: "Quite simply, this time, he [Lutwidge] had got it wrong".[5]

However, it was not his work, but his untimely and grisly end, met in the course of his work which he was still continuing in his eighth decade, which may assure Lutwidge of the attention of posterity. The account in the *Journal of Mental Science* of July 1873 gives the details:

> Our readers will have seen with deep regret the announcement of the death of Mr. R. W. S. Lutwidge, who was so long connected with the Lunacy Board – first as secretary to the Commissioners, and afterwards as a Commissioner. While visiting Fisherton House Asylum [in Salisbury], in company with Mr. Wilkes, he was suddenly attacked by a patient, who struck him violently on the temple with a nail, which had evidently been concealed and prepared for the purpose of inflicting injury on some one. An attack of paralysis followed, which ended fatally at Salisbury. Mr.

Lutwidge was 72 years of age, so that it was not probable that, in the natural course of events, he would have continued to perform his active duties as a Commissioner for many more years; but it is beyond measure sad that a long and useful life should have been brought to an end in so distressing a manner. Mr. Lutwidge will be generally regretted by those who were brought in contact with him in his official capacity, and who could not fail to appreciate the courteous and genial manners of a kind-hearted gentleman. It must needs be that accidents happen from time to time in asylums; indeed, the marvel is that they are not more numerous than they are, when we consider how many irresponsible beings, danger-ous to themselves or to others, are collected in them. An event of this kind is well calculated to make us appreciate more justly than we perhaps commonly do the trials, the endurance, and the unwelcome work of those attendants upon the insane who are in constant intercourse with them, and from whom we demand a long-suffering and a gentleness that are more than human.[7]

The attack occurred on 21st May, and Lutwidge died a week later. The events were also noted in the *British Medical Journal*, in the issue of 7th June 1873:

Mr. R. S. [sic] Lutwidge, Commissioner in Lunacy, has succumbed to the injuries inflicted on him by a criminal lunatic, who stabbed him in the temple with a nail on the 21st instant, as he was inspecting the Fisherton House Criminal Lunatic Asylum, in company with Mr. J. Wilkes, also a Commissioner in Lunacy. (*BMJ* 1873;1:651).

According to the account in the *Hampshire Advertiser* newspaper of the inquest held on 29th May, the perpetrator was one William M'Kave who, according to Dr. Corbin Finch, one of the asylum's owners, "had been in the asylum twenty years last December. He was a noisy, irritable, discontented man, but was not considered a dangerous lunatic. He had a delusion that some woman with whom he had cohabited constantly haunted him in the asylum. He was always complaining whenever the inspectors or others went into the ward".[8]

In his Presidential Address to the members of the Medico-Psychological Association delivered at the Royal College of Physicians in London on 6th August 1873, Harrington Tuke noted that:

Since our last yearly meeting we have lost a friend, who, although not a member of the Society nor of our profession, had been long engaged in the work in which we are still hopefully toiling. For more than thirty years he acted as Secretary to the Commissioners in Lunacy, and afterwards as Commissioner; and during the tenure of this important office he lost his useful life in the performance of his duty. I am sure you will feel, that as your President, I am right to pay my and your tribute of respect to the memory of Mr. Lutwidge.[9]

For Carrollians, the obvious question is whether R.W.S. Lutwidge had any influence on his nephew or on his written works? Certainly C.L. Dodgson visited his uncle on the day after the attack and was instrumental in arranging the attendance of the eminent physician Sir James Paget (the whole story has been told by Geoffrey Budworth[10]). Perhaps reassured by Paget's hopeful prognosis, Dodgson then left Salisbury, only to return shortly after Lutwidge's death a week later. He also attended the funeral in London on 3rd June.

As regards Carroll's work, the answer to the question of any putative influence of Lutwidge is unequivocally in the affirmative. Specifically, in *The Hunting of the Snark* wherein Carroll mentions (Fit 3, stanza 6, line 1), in lines spoken by The Baker, "A dear uncle of mine (after whom I was named)". The poem was first published in 1876, three years after Lutwidge's death, but it was not until 2004 that this identification was suggested by Torrey and Miller.[11] It has become incorporated into Martin Gardner's annotated *Hunting of the Snark*,[12] and Torrey and Miller have also revisited the issue.[13] Gardner also points out that other passages "strengthen the view that Carroll was satirizing himself in the person of the Baker".

If he is known at all now, Lutwidge is perhaps most remembered for his work in photography, an interest shared with his nephew.

Acknowledgement

Unpublished manuscript, Spring 2024.

References

1. *Biographies of Legal Lunacy Commissioners and Secretaries 1832–1912.* http://studymore.org.uk/6biol.htm (accessed 19/03/2024)
2. *Report of the Committee of Visitors of the Bedford Lunatic Asylum, for the year ending the 31st December, 1859.* Bedford: W.C. Grey, 1860: 9–10.
3. Cashman B. *A Proper House. Bedford Lunatic Asylum: 1812–1860.* Bedford: North Bedfordshire Health Authority, 1992 ["Lutteridge": 127, 134; "W.S. Lutwidge": 115, 116].
4. *Report of the Committee of Visitors and of the Medical Superintendent of the West Riding Pauper Lunatic Asylum for the year 1870.* Wakefield: B.W. Allen, 1871: 9–15.
5. *Report of the Committee of Visitors and of the Medical Superintendent of the West Riding Pauper Lunatic Asylum for the year 1871.* Wakefield: B.W. Allen, 1872: 7–14.

6. Scrimgeour D. *Proper people. Early asylum life in the words of those who were there*. York: York Publishing, 2015: 253–254.
7. Anon. The late Mr. Lutwidge. *J Ment Sci* 1873–1874; 19 (July 1873): 264–265.
8. *Hampshire Advertiser* 31st May 1873, p.7 (Murder of a Lunacy Commissioner).
9. Harrington Tuke T. The Medico-Psychological Association. The President's Address for 1873. *J Ment Sci* 1873–1874; 19 (October 1873): 327–340 [quote at 328].
10. Budworth G. The killing of Skeffington Lutwidge. *The Carrollian* 2010; 26: 52–55.
11. Torrey EF, Miller J. The capture of the Snark. *Knight Letter* 2004; 73: 21–25.
12. Gardner M (ed.). *The annotated Hunting of the Snark. The definitive edition*. New York: WW Norton, 2006: xxiv-xxv, 37–38.
13. Torrey EF, Miller J. Violence and mental illness: what Lewis Carroll had to say. *Schizophrenia Res* 2014; 160: 33–34.

John Charles Bucknill (1817–1897): pioneer in neurology?

John Charles Bucknill was not a neurologist as currently understood, but an alienist or psychiatrist. Nevertheless, it is the argument of this paper that he merits designation as a "Pioneer in Neurology" for his contributions to the beginnings of *Brain: a journal of neurology*, one of the most eminent journals in the field over the past 150 years. Of the founding editors of *Brain*, John Hughlings Jackson (1835–1911) [14] and David Ferrier (1843–1928) [11] are familiar names to neurologists, and James Crichton-Browne (1840–1938), although an alienist, has been included in the *Journal of Neurology* Pioneers in Neurology series [3]. Evidently then, Bucknill is the least well-known of *Brain*'s founding quadrumvirate, at least in neurological circles.

Bucknill's biography has been recounted, *qua* alienist [6,12] and, much more briefly, in his role at *Brain* [1,5]. After training at University College London, he was appointed aged twenty-six as superintendent of the newly opened Devon County Lunatic Asylum at Exminster, a village just south of the city of Exeter. During his eighteen years there, he pioneered methods of non-restraint and when overcrowding became an issue (as it did for all county asylums in this era) he experimented with housing chronic patients in small houses both in and beyond the asylum grounds [10].

Bucknill was a prolific writer. He co-authored, with Daniel Hack Tuke (1827–1895), a physician at York Retreat, the significant textbook, *A Manual of Psychological Medicine* (1858), in which his contribution dealt with the diagnosis, pathology and treatment of insanity [2]. Perhaps most significantly for his subsequent role in the history of neurology, he was the first editor of the *Asylum Journal of Medical Science*, official journal of the Association of Medical Officers of Asylums and Hospitals for the Insane. Commenced in 1853, Bucknill served as editor until 1862, renaming it the *Journal of Mental Science* in 1858 (it became the *British Journal of Psychiatry* in 1963) [6].

As befitting an erudite gentleman physician, he took an interest in the works of Shakespeare, publishing books on *The Psychology of Shakespeare* (1859) and *The Medical Knowledge of Shakespeare* (1860). He became a Fellow of the Royal College of Physicians (RCP) of London in 1859 and of the Royal Society in 1866. Between 1862 and 1875 he was Lord Chancellor's Visitor in Lunacy, a public office with the remit to inspect care and treatment of patients deemed insane by the Court of Chancery. He was Lumleian lecturer at the RCP in 1878 ("Habitual drunkards and insane drunkards"), long before Hughlings Jackson (1890) and Ferrier (1906) received this honour.

The origins of *Brain* are obscure; apparently no records exist for its first 25 years of operation. Some contend that Crichton-Browne was the principal moving force behind its inception since, as superintendent of the West Riding Asylum at Wakefield, he had previously edited the *West Riding Lunatic Asylum Medical Reports* (*WRLAMR*) between 1871–1876. Both Ferrier and Hughlings Jackson made significant contributions to *WRLAMR* [7], Ferrier's being based on his experimental researches commenced at the asylum in 1873 [8]. Others have suggested Ferrier was key to *Brain*'s inauguration: according to Sherrington "it was Ferrier who urged that the work which the Reports [*WRLAMR*] had begun, should be in some form continued. It then came to be agreed that a "Neurological Journal" should be started in London, and thus "Brain" was launched" [13]. Henson [5] noted that Bucknill was the senior editor, and certainly this was true based on year of birth, by nearly twenty years, but that Crichton Browne was the "leading spirit".

How had Bucknill come to be associated with this group, and hence with the beginnings of *Brain*? Such was the porosity of evolving professional boundaries in the late 19th century that diseases now deemed "neurological" would inevitably have been dealt with by alienists (for example epilepsy) as well as by those developing the specialty of neurology. Although he did not publish in *WRLAMR*, Bucknill lectured at Wakefield Asylum at the annual meeting, or *conversazione*, of 20th November 1874 ("Responsibility for Homicide"). His eminence in his field, and his evident commitment to "physical pathology and the direct application of scientific medicine in understanding insanity" [12] marked him as like-minded with the other editors, such that he could endorse the effective "manifesto" of *Brain* (published in the journal *Mind* 1878;3:295):

> "The Journal will ... include in its scope all that relates to the anatomy, physiology, pathology and therapeutics of the Nervous System. The functions and diseases of the nervous system will be discussed both in their physiological and psychological aspects; but mental phenomena will be treated only in correlation with their anatomical substrata, and mental disease will be investigated as far as possible by the methods applicable to nervous diseases in general".

Bucknill's extensive prior editorial experience with the *Journal of Mental Science* (it has been estimated that he was responsible for 40–45% of the content in the first three volumes [12]) was also undoubtedly a factor in his recruitment.

Certainly Bucknill was an assiduous contributor to the early volumes of *Brain*. He published in the "Critical Digests and Notices of Books" section of the journal in the inaugural issue of April 1878 (as did Ferrier) and continued to do so until 1885 (in all, 15 such publications). Although there were more substantive papers – "The late Lord Chief Justice of England on Lunacy" in 1881; "Dean Swift's disease" and "The plea of insanity in the case of Charles Julius Guiteau" in 1882 – he did not publish any original clinical or experimental work in *Brain*, unlike Crichton-Browne, Hughlings Jackson and Ferrier [7]. His contributions tailed off after the appointment of Armand de Watteville (1846–1925) as "acting editor" of *Brain* in 1884 [9].

Whatever his exact commitments to *Brain* after the mid-1880s, Bucknill still moved in neurological circles. He was a founder member of the Neurological Society of London in 1886, serving on the council with Ferrier; Hughlings Jackson was president, Crichton-Browne was one of the two vice-presidents. Undoubtedly, then, the quadrumvirate were involved in the adoption of *Brain* as the official journal of the Neurological Society in 1887.

Bucknill's name is remembered at Exeter within the Bucknill Centre in Wonford House Hospital and also in Northernhay Gardens where the Volunteer Force of Great Britain, a corps of citizen-soldiers [4], later to become The Territorial Army, is commemorated on a monument that includes his carved image. Thereon it is noted that "In recognition of his services to the Volunteer Movement, the Honour of Knighthood was conferred" in 1894, rather than for any of his clinical work.

Acknowledgement

Adapted and extended from: Larner AJ, Gardner-Thorpe C. John Charles Bucknill (1817–1897). *J Neurol* 2023;270:4154–4155.

References

1. Anon (1978) One hundred years ago. Practitioner 220:984.
2. Beveridge A (1998) The odd couple: the partnership of J.C. Bucknill and D.H. Tuke. Psychiatr Bull 22:52–56
3. Cambiaghi M (2019) James Crichton-Browne (1840–1938). J Neurol 266:1819–1820
4. Clapham C (1897) Sir John Charles Bucknill, M.D., F.R.C.P., F.R.S., Citizen-soldier and Psychologist. J Ment Sci 43:885–889
5. Henson RA (1978) The editors of *Brain*. Practitioner 221:639–644
6. Langley GE (1980) Sir John Charles Bucknill 1817–1897: our founder. Br J Psychiatry 137:105–110
7. Larner AJ (2023) The *West Riding Lunatic Asylum Medical Reports* – the precursor of *Brain*? Brain 146:4437–4445.
8. Larner AJ (2023) A month in the country: the sesquicentenary of David

Ferrier's classical cerebral localisation researches of 1873. J R Coll Physicians Edinb 52:128–131

9. Larner AJ, Triarhou LC (2025) Armand de Watteville (1846–1925). J Neurol 272:136.

10. Morgan N (1990) Against the tide at Exmouth: J.C. Bucknill 1817–1897. South West Psychiatry 4:73–76

11. Sandrone S, Zanin E (2014) David Ferrier (1843–1928). J Neurol 261:1247–1248

12. Scull A, Mackenzie C, Hervey N (1996) Masters of Bedlam. The transformation of the mad-doctoring trade. Princeton: Princeton University Press; 187–225

13. Sherrington CS (1928) Sir David Ferrier, 1843–1928. Proc R Soc Lond B Biol Sci 103:viii-xvi

14. Swash M (2005) John Hughlings Jackson (1835–1911). J Neurol 252:745–746

Ignaz Philipp Semmelweis (1818–1865)

In the lying-in hospitals of nineteenth century Europe, puerperal sepsis or childbed fever was an occupational hazard for women in labour. Mortality rates of 1 in 6 were not unusual, occasionally 1 in 3 would die, and in bad epidemics more than half of the women would not surivive their accouchement. The only remedy in such a situation was to close the hospital until the epidemic had passed.

Most women gave birth at home, but for unmarried mothers, disowned by their families, there was a real prospect of giving birth in the streets. The large numbers of such women in Vienna had prompted Empress Marie Therese to give money for the operation of two gratis maternity clinics at the general hospital to which any woman would be admitted with no questions asked. The First Clinic of the lying-in division was administered by doctors and medical students, the Second Clinic was run by midwives.

Such was the terror of childbed fever, which only occurred to any extent in the hospital, that many women still preferred to deliver their children in the streets rather than risk confinement in the hospital.

Theories as to the aetiology of puerperal sepsis were legion: it was the result of a miasma, of cosmic-telluric influences, of wounded modesty as a result of the frequent physical examinations, of poor hospital ventilation, of suppression of the lochia, of a milk fever, an inevitable condition following pregnancy, and so on. All authorities were agreed that it was incurable. Such a fatalistic attitude toward the suffering of so many women did not satisfy a young obstetrical assistant in the Vienna General Hospital in 1844. Ignaz Philipp Semmelweis, a Hungarian, and therefore looked down on as a provincial boor by the haughty Imperial Viennese, had originally come to the university to read law. Dragged along to a post-mortem as a dare by medical students he became so entirely engrossed that he decided that medicine was his true vocation. As a student he became well-known for interrupting lectures to ask searching questions which did not endear him to certain professors but won the respect of others, such as Karl Rokitansky, professor of pathology and prosector at the Vienna General Hospital, and Jakob Kolletschka, professor of medico-legal jurisprudence.

Appointed to an assistant's post in the First Obstetrical clinic, Semmelweis was appalled by the suffering he witnessed on the wards. The director of the clinic was Joseph Klein, a man who cared only for order in his wards and who, like many, was dependent for his position at the hospital on powerful friends at the Imperial court. He had instituted the use of the cadaver for the teaching of obstetrics so replacing the "phantom," a model of wood and leather, used by his predecessor. He ascribed puerperal sepsis to a miasma, for which there was no treatment, and he did not respond enthusiastically to Semmelweis's attempts to find a remedy.

Semmelweis grew familiar with puerperal sepsis by his work on the ward and by the many dissections he performed, along with Rokitansky and Kolletschka, before attending to his patients each morning. Symptomatically it consisted of shivering and acute pain, radiating from the uterus, starting from the second to the fourth day of confinement. The pain gradually extended to all over the abdomen, with suppression of lochia and milk, tachycardia, furred tongue, dyspnoea and drawing up of the knees. The form and intensity of the symptoms was very variable between cases, but fever was the cardinal sign. Pathologically too the picture was varied with endometritis, peritonitis, phlebitis, meningitis, pericarditis, pleurisy and lymphangitis, though not all were always present. Dissection complete he would walk to the ward and examine all the women in labour, pausing only to wipe his hands on a towel or the lapels of his coat, as was customary, then dipping his fingers in lard to facilitate examination.

A most intriguing finding, gleaned from analysis of the hospital records, was that the mortality rate in the First Clinic was three times that in the Second Clinic. Traditionally this was explained either by localization of the miasma only over the First Clinic, or by the gentler examinations performed by the midwives. Further perusal of the records of the clinic showed Semmelweis that the death rate had been lower before Klein became director, and that the longer the labour the greater the chance of puerperal fever.

Deterioration of his relationship with Klein caused Semmelweis to be temporarily dismissed in 1846, and on his return he was surprised to find that the death rate had declined in his absence. Klein was apt to blame him for this because he was a foreigner: commissions appointed to investigate the previous outbreaks had blamed the soaring death rate on the presence of foreign students.

The death of Kolletschka was a severe blow to Semmelweis; while demonstrating on a cadaver, he had been accidentally cut by a careless student and had subsequently died of cadaveric poisoning. The findings at post-mortem were reported as peritonitis, pleurisy, lymphangitis, meningitis and pericarditis. Semmelweis realised that these were exactly the same as the findings in those dying of puerperal sepsis. Indeed it was known that men could very occasionally die of "puerperal" sepsis, but the link between these findings and putrefying organic matter had never been made. Semmelweis realised that his industry in the dissecting room had inadvertently condemned many women, since it was his practice to examine the women directly afterwards. His temporary replacement had not dissected, and thus had not carried infected material to the women. Similarly the midwives did not dissect, hence the lower mortality in the Second Clinic. Before Klein's arrival, obstetrics were taught on the phantom rather than the cadaver, the obvious source of infective material. The longer a woman's labour the more times she was examined and so the greater the chance of her being infected.

On making this discovery, Semmelweis instantly instituted washing with soap and water and with chlorine solution, known to have antiseptic properties, before examining the women. Such innovations did not please Klein who fretted about the cost of the materials, nor the students who thought it humiliating to have to wash and have their hands inspected, a routine which the midwives had tolerated for many years. Nonetheless, Semmelweis persisted and the death rate began to decline dramatically, actually falling below that in the Second Clinic in 1848, and in two months there were no deaths at all. By dint of the occasional deaths that did occur, Semmelweis was able to show that any putrid organic material could cause sepsis, e.g. from a medullary sarcoma of the uterus, or the foul discharge from a leg ulcer, or such matter on a sheet. He rigidly enforced cleanliness in the clinic despite the recalcitrance of the students.

To his chagrin, the medical hierarchy received his discovery with amusement, comforting themselves in the belief that puerperal sepsis was inevitable and incurable. However, Semmelweis was championed by certain of the academics: Joseph Skoda, Karl Rokitansky, and Ferdinand Hebra who published two accounts of the results in the prestigious Vienna Medical Society Journal in 1847 and 1848. However, despite this support, reaction was generally hostile, and although Simpson wrote from London claiming that the contagiousness of puerperal sepsis was a British idea, he failed to understand the implications of Semmelweis's work for its prophylaxis.

Unable to get a post as a lecturer which would enable him to spread the doctrine, Semmelweis returned to his home town of Pesth where he was appointed professor of theoretical and practical midwifery. In the minuscule clinic there he achieved in 1857 the incredible feat of a whole year without a single death due to childbed fever. Still he was ignored or worse still mocked – the great Virchow, then the oracle of Middle Europe, called him the "Pesth Fool" (so much for his liberalism). Semmelweis tried to convince his critics by experimentation: putrid material inoculated into the uterus of a rat caused exactly the same pathological manifestations as in the women; the miasma theory was answered by showing that of two rats in a cage, one infected and the other not, only the infected one died – it was not feasible that a miasmatic cloud selectively hover over one rat and not the other.

When this approach failed Semmelweis attempted to convince his contemporaries of the merit of his doctrine by writing a book on the aetiology and treatment of puerperal sepsis but little notice was taken. Finally worn out by his efforts he was committed to an asylum and died there in 1865.

Many claims of precedence over Semmelweis for being the first to discover the contagious nature of puerperal sepsis have been made, there being a particularly strong lobby on behalf of Oliver Wendell Holmes in the USA. Undoubtedly he did publish an essay on the subject in 1843 but unlike Semmelweis he failed to identify a necessary cause for all cases of puerperal fever. Semmelweis's unique contribution was to realise that there was a necessary and therefore treatable cause for all cases of childbed fever without having to resort to the metaphysics of the miasma. He also observed that the puerperal state was not a necessary condition for the inception of the disease, as it could be contracted during delivery or even during pregnancy with fatal results. Essentially Semmelweis conducted an epidemiological study from which he was able to conclude that all cases of puerperal sepsis had a common cause, and this many years before the identification of specific infective agents – it is now known that beta-haemolytic streptococci are usually responsible for such pyaemic conditions. The sine qua non of his aetiological characterisation was the resorption of decaying animal-organic matter, and his doctrine gave not only practical advice for avoiding some cases of puerperal fever but a complete explanatory scientific theory.

Addendum (2023)

At the original time of writing (1985), I was unaware of the "Semmelweis reflex" or "Semmelweis effect" – the tendency to reject reflexively any new knowledge because it conflicts with or frankly contradicts existing or established norms or paradigms.

Acknowledgement

Adapted from: Larner AJ. Ignaz Philipp Semmelweis. *Oxford Medical School Gazette* 1985;36(2):5–7. This was my very first printed piece, written when I was a medical student at the University of Oxford Medical School (1984–1987).

References

Codell Carter K. Semmelweis and his predecessors. *Medical History* 1981; 25: 57–72.
Dawson PM. Semmelweis, an interpretation. *Ann Med Hist* 1924; 6: 258–279.

McIntosh Marshall C. Semmelweis. Some brief glimpses of his life and work. *Sphincter* 1943; 6(2): 9–14.

Semmelweis IP. *Die Aetiologie, der Begriff und die Prophylaxis des Kindbettfiebers.* 1861.

Sinclair WJ. *Semmelweis. His life and his doctrine. A chapter in the history of medicine.* Manchester: Manchester University Press, 1909.

Thompson M. *The cry and the covenant.* London: William Heinemann, 1951.

John Hughlings Jackson (1835–1911): an addition to his published writings?

In his biography of John Hughlings Jackson, Samuel Greenblatt noted, in the context of the bibliography of Jackson's published papers, numbering more than 500, that "Doubtless there are still more out there".[1] Briefly, I thought I had found one, and after further investigation this may still be the case. The story is as follows.

In the *Transactions of the Medical Society of London* for 1891, under the heading "CASE OF TREADLER'S CRAMP. By J. HUGHLINGS JACKSON, M.D., F.R.S.", this brief note appeared:

> Dr. RIVERS showed for Dr. Hughlings Jackson a case of treadler's cramp occurring in a man who, after having been a hand-loom weaver for thirty years, began to make mistakes in his work owing to defective treadling with his right leg (the one principally used); later the right leg became lame, and after using the left leg for some years this became weak, rendering him unable to follow his occupation. The spasm occurred at the commencement of the flexion movement which accompanied the upward motion of the treadle, the extension or downward movement being well performed. The spasm was of the combined movement of the hip and knee, each joint being moved freely by itself. The difficulty was referred by the patient to the gluteal region, and both the gluteal and hamstring muscles on the right side showed decided diminution of faradic and galvanic irritability. The right leg was held stiffly in walking, the case thus agreeing with other occupation spasms in which large movements were concerned, and in which the affected limb was more or less generally disabled.[2] [capitals in original].

As Greenblatt points out, most of Hughlings Jackson's papers "were originally given at meetings of medical organizations"[1] of which there were many in late nineteenth-century London. These oral papers were then reported in the weekly medical press, sometimes two, three or even four versions appearing in the different journals, not only the *Lancet* and the *British Medical Journal* but also the *Medical Times and Gazette* and the *Medical Press and Circular*. This appears to be borne out for the case of treadler's cramp.

There are two substantial published bibliographies of Hughlings Jackson's work: the Catalogue Raisonné of York & Steinberg (2006) and Greenblatt's "Published writings of John Hughlings Jackson" (2022). Consulting these sources for the year 1891,[3,4] one finds that the case of treadler's cramp was reported in the *Lancet* and in *Brain* (York & Steinberg items [91–01] and [91–06]). The *Lancet* report (identical wording to that given above) related to a meeting which took place at the Medical Society of London on 16th February.[5] However, the original publication in the *Transactions of the Medical Society of London* appears in neither bibliography.

Why this oversight? Why did these distinguished authors not think to access the original presentation, rather than simply report thereof? One possible explanation might be that these authors were unaware of this relatively obscure journal, but more likely, I think, the journal may have been inaccessible rather than unknown to them. (I saw this journal on a pre-arranged visit to the Medical Society of London, although it is available through Internet Archive.)

What can one make of the actual case report? Irrespective of the well-recognised shortcomings of attempted retrospective diagnosis, I suspect that many neurologists will want to venture a diagnostic or differential diagnostic opinion, notwithstanding the paucity of clinical information (no examination!). My reading, for what it is worth, is that the 30–year history of repetitive flexion-extension movement might make compressive lumbosacral radiculopathies in the context of degenerative spinal disease the most likely diagnosis; this might also perhaps account for the "diminution of faradic and galvanic irritability" in the gluteal and hamstring muscles. However, the mention of spasm and of stiffness in the leg may perhaps suggest a more proximally located (i.e. central) disorder: is this a form of occupational or task-specific dystonia, *avant le nom*?

Luckily, as in any typical grand round presentation, further clinical information is available! Unlike the *Lancet* report, which is identical to the *Transactions of the Medical Society of London* account, the *Brain* report is quite different. Indeed, it is related to a different meeting, that of the Neurological Society (of London) held on 5th March 1891, and Jackson's name does not appear on the by-line.[6] Now we are given details of the man's age (56) and initials (J.M.), and some examination findings: "The tendon jerks are equal and not exaggerated" and the right glutei and hamstring muscles are wasted compared to the left. Moreover:

the flexion of the limb when treadling is performed with great difficulty, as if some resistance were being overcome, the thigh becoming inverted during the process.

Could this resistance be involuntary co-contraction of agonist and antagonist muscles? Could the thigh inversion be dystonic posturing?

The spasm can be lessened by supporting the lower end of the thigh, and especially when any pressure is exerted on the popliteal space. ... whether in the present case the improvement is due to any pressure on the nerve I have not been able to determine, but am inclined to attribute it solely to support of the limb.

Could this be a sensory trick which relieves a dystonic posture?

The patient walks leaning forward and using the right leg very stiffly. He goes upstairs with difficulty; downstairs easily. That the gait should be affected is in accordance with ... [the] observation that, while in an occupation spasm, like writer's cramp, in which the movements concerned are fine, the affection is usually, though not invariably, limited to the act of writing; in those in which the movements are large ... the limb suffers for modes of action other than that of the occupation. Since both walking and going upstairs involve flexion of the limb similar to that which occurs in treadling, it might be expected that they would suffer in this case.

The comparison here with writer's cramp, another "occupation spasm", is of note, although the appearance of symptoms when walking as well as when treadling may be more in keeping with a task-specific dystonia. Rivers reported Hughlings Jackson's view of these cases as follows:

He considers that the affections known as occupation spasms are due to defective action of some elements of the spinal centres, or their homologues higher up.

Whatever the diagnosis in this patient may have been, the attempted formulation presented here may illustrate how the clinical approach to cases changes over time, not merely in terms of investigations available but conceptually.

York & Steinberg stated that the "Dr. Rivers" by whom the case was presented on behalf of Hughlings Jackson, at both the Medical Society of London and the Neurological Society, was W.H.R. Rivers (1864–1922). Indeed, this is the name which appears on the by-line of the *Brain* paper.[6] Rivers is perhaps best known to posterity for his work with patients suffering from shell-shock during the First World War, but at this early stage in his career he was house physician at the National Hospital for the Paralysed and Epileptic at Queen Square (although mentioned only in passing in this capacity in Shorvon & Compston's history of the National[7]). It was apparently at this time that Rivers also met and became friends with another physician from the London Hospital, Henry Head, with whom he later (1903–1907) collaborated in a famous experiment on the consequences of nerve division, Head being the experimental subject.[8,9]

Postscript

Some months after writing this piece, it came to my notice that reference to "'Case of treadler's cramp' *Trans. Med. Soc.*, xiv., 1891, 439." did appear in the bibliography of Hughlings Jackson's papers prepared by Sir William Broadbent in his 1903 paper on Jackson. This was the 3rd Hughlings Jackson Lecture held under the auspices of the Neurological Society of the United Kingdom (as it had been renamed in 1903), delivered on 5th November 1903 and subsequently published in *Brain*.[10] That being the case, the absence of this paper from the bibliographic works of York & Steinberg and of Greenblatt is all the more mysterious. (Henry Head's "Bibliography of papers on affections of speech by Dr. Hughlings Jackson arranged chronologically" published in *Brain* 1915;38:187–190 is not relevant here.)

Acknowledgements

Original manuscript, 28th April 2024; postscript 24th August 2024. Original manuscript published *Adv Clin Neurosci Rehabil* 2024; 23 (1): 24-25.

References

1. Greenblatt SH. *John Hughlings Jackson. Clinical neurology, evolution, and Victorian brain science.* Oxford: Oxford University Press, 2022: 7.
2. Jackson JH. Case of treadler's cramp. *Trans Med Soc Lond* 1891; 14: 439.
3. York GK, Steinberg DA. An introduction to the life and work of John Hughlings Jackson with a catalogue raisonné of his writings. *Med Hist Suppl* 2006; 26: 121.
4. Op. cit., ref. 1: 496–7.
5. Medical Society of London. *Lancet* 1891; 1(3521): 433–5 (21st February) [case at 434].
6. Rivers WHR. A case of treadler's cramp. *Brain* 1891; 14 (1): 110–1.
7. Shorvon S, Compston A. *Queen Square. A history of the National Hospital and its Institute of Neurology.* Cambridge: Cambridge University Press, 2019: 342.
8. Rivers WHR, Head H. A human experiment in nerve division. *Brain* 1908; 31 (3): 332–450.
9. Jacyna LS. *Medicine and modernism: A biography of Henry Head.* Pittsburgh: University of Pittsburgh Press, 2016: 125–30.
10 Broadbent W. Hughlings Jackson as pioneer in nervous physiology and pathology. *Brain* 1903; 26(3): 305–66 [at 365].

Théodule-Armand Ribot (1839–1916): first report of transient global amnesia?

Théodule-Armand Ribot (1839–1916) is probably best remembered for his "law of regression of memories", enunciated in his 1881 monograph *Les maladies de la Mémoire* (*Diseases of memory*) which holds that more recent memories are forgotten before older memories.[1] Certainly this temporal gradient is typically encountered in the amnesia of Alzheimer's disease.

Some recent authors have claimed that Ribot described the syndrome of transient global amnesia (TGA) in his monograph. For example, Daniel states that Ribot "described transient amnestic states suggestive of TGA" in his 1881 work,[2] and this claim has been repeated by other authors writing on TGA,[3] but likewise eschewing quotation or precise page citation from Ribot's book.

If true, these claims would represent a 19th century account of TGA, predating the earliest generally accepted account, that of Benon in 1909,[4] as documented by Pearce and Bogousslavsky.[5]

To try to ascertain whether or not Ribot did describe TGA, I consulted the English translation of his book made by William Huntington Smith and published in New York in 1882.

Although Ribot certainly addresses the subject of temporary amnesia, as compared with periodic and progressive amnesia, I find no compelling account of TGA. The most suggestive is simply a citation of a case previously presented in 1835 by "Kömpfen",[6] parts of which are reproduced here:

"I must give a few details, apparently insignificant of themselves, but worth knowing, since they relate to a remarkable phenomenon. During the latter part of November, an officer of my regiment had his left foot injured by the pressure of an ill-fitting boot. On the 30th of November he went to Versailles to meet his brother. He dined there, returning to Paris the same night, and, on entering his lodgings, found a letter from his father on the mantel-piece. We now come to the important point. On the first of December this officer was at the riding-school, and, his horse falling, he was thrown, striking upon the right side of his body, and particularly upon the right parietal. The shock was followed by a slight syncope. On coming to himself, he remounted "to drive off a little giddiness," and continued his lesson for three quarters of an hour with much assiduity. From time to time, however, he kept saying to the riding-master, "I have been dreaming. What has happened to me?" He was finally taken home. Living in the same house with the patient, I was immediately called in. He was standing, recognized me and greeted me as usual saying, "I seem to have been dreaming. What has happened to me?" His speech is natural, he replies readily to all questions and complains only of a confused feeling in the head.

"Notwithstanding my inquiries, and those of the riding-master, and of his servant, he remembers neither the injury to his foot, nor his journey to Versailles, nor going out in the morning, nor the orders he gave on going out, nor his fall, nor what followed. He recognizes everyone, calls each visitor by his name, and knows his position by officer. I have not allowed an hour to pass without examining the patient. Each time that I go back he believes that I have come for the first time. He remembers nothing of the prescribed remedies administered (foot-bath, rubbing, etc.). In a word, nothing exists for him except the action of the moment.

"Six hours after the accident ... the patient takes cognizance of the reply already made so many times, "You fell from your horse!"

"Eight hours after the accident ... the patient remembers to have seen me once before.

"Two hours and a half later ... the patient no longer forgets what is said to him. He remembers distinctly the injury to his foot. He begins also to recall his visit to Versailles yesterday, but so indistinctly that he says if any one were to affirm positively to the contrary he would be disposed to believe him. However, the memory continuing to return, by night he became firmly convinced that he had been to Versailles. But here the progress of recollection ceased for the day. He went to bed without remembering what he had done at Versailles, how he had returned to Paris, of the receipt of his father's letter.

"December 2nd – after a night of tranquil sleep, he remembers on awakening what he did at Versailles, how he came back, and that he found a letter from his father on the mantel-piece. But of all that he saw or heard on the 1st of December, before his fall, he is still ignorant to-day – that is to say, he has no knowledge of the events in question save from the testimony of others."

To be sure, if one may indulge in the anachronistic, retrospective, application of the widely accepted clinical diagnostic criteria for TGA proposed by Hodges and Warlow in 1990,[7] some appear to be definitely fulfilled in this account, viz.: the attack was witnessed and information made available from a capable observer (I presume a military doctor) who was present for most of the attack; there was clear-cut anterograde amnesia during the attack; and the attack resolved within 24 hours. Other criteria seem likely to have been fulfilled, viz.: there was no report of obvious clouding of consciousness or loss of personal identity, and from the given account the cognitive impairment seemed to be limited to amnesia (i.e. no aphasia, apraxia); there were no accompanying focal neurological symptoms during the attack and no significant neurological signs afterwards; and epileptic features were absent. However, the seventh criterion is not fulfilled, viz.: patients with recent head injury are excluded from a diagnosis of TGA. The report could be simply a case of post-traumatic amnesia.

Although Ribot states of this case that "I transcribe it almost entire", consulting the original article gives some additional information, such as the fact that the patient was 28 years old, an age at which TGA is unlikely to occur.

Thus, to answer the question posed by the title of this piece, Ribot definitely did not describe TGA in the nineteenth century. Certainly Koempfen's 1835 case description is that of a transient amnesia which might be deemed "suggestive", but certainly not diagnostic, of TGA as now understood. Hence Benon's 1909 case currently remains the earliest convincing description to my knowledge.

This is not to say, of course, that TGA did not occur before the 20th century: absence of evidence is not equivalent to evidence of absence. The ontological challenge to the persistence of disease over historical time,[8] suggesting as it does in this situation that mechanisms of mnestic hippocampal function have changed, is simply not credible.

Acknowledgement

Adapted from: Larner AJ. Did Ribot describe transient global amnesia in the nineteenth century? *Cortex* 2021;138:38–39.

References

1. Ribot, Th. (1882). *Diseases of memory: an essay in the positive psychology.* New York: D Appleton and Company. https://archive.org/stream/cu31924031165719?ref=ol#page/n39/mode/2up

2. Daniel, B.T. (2012). *Transient global amnesia.* Print version and ebook: Amazon.

3. Foss-Skiftesvik, J., Snoer, A.H., Wagner, A., & Hauerberg, J. (2015). Transient global amnesia after cerebral angiography still occurs: case report and literature review. *Radiology Case Reports, 9*, 988. doi: 10.2484/rcr.v9i4.988

4. Benon, R. (1909). Les ictus amnésiques dans les démences "organiques". *Ann Méd Psychol, 67*, 207–219.

5. Pearce, J.M.S., & Bogousslavsky, J. (2009). "Les ictus amnésiques" and transient global amnesia. *European Neurology, 62*, 188–192. doi: 10.1159/000228263

6. Koempfen, M. (1835). Observation sur un cas de perte de mémoire. *Mémoires de l'Academie Nationale de Médecine, 4*, 489–494. https://gallica.bnf.fr/ark:/12148/bpt6k6361350t/f507.item

7. Hodges, J.R., & Warlow, C.P. (1990). Syndromes of transient amnesia: towards a classification. A study of 153 cases. *Journal of Neurology, Neurosurgery and Psychiatry*, 53, 834–843. doi: 10.1136/jnnp.53.10.834

8. Muramoto, O. (2014). Retrospective diagnosis of a famous historical figure: ontological, epistemic, and ethical considerations. *Philosophy, Ethics, and Humanities in Medicine*, 9: 10. doi: 10.1186/1747–5341–9–10

James Crichton-Browne (1840–1938) and Dickens

The first half of the nineteenth century witnessed a programme of asylum building for the care of the insane in England. This was facilitated by passage of the County Asylum Acts of 1808 and 1845, the first a permissive discretionary act enabling local authorities to provide suitable accommodation for those paupers committed as insane, the latter a compulsory act requiring such provision. These changes in the social fabric were unlikely to have eluded Charles Dickens's gaze, related as they were to prisons and workhouses wherein many individuals with mental health problems were inappropriately detained.

It is known that Dickens visited St. Luke's Asylum in London on Boxing Day 1851,[1] and Lancaster Asylum in September 1857 during his tour of the North with Wilkie Collins.[2] Just a month before the latter visit, Dickens had published a commentary following a visit to Bethlem Hospital, the proverbial Bedlam, in *Household Words*,[3] and later in the same year in his article on the asylum reformer Dr John Conolly (1794–1866)[4] he noted that Dr Samuel Gaskell, brother-in-law of Elizabeth Gaskell, had adopted the system of non-restraint in the Asylum at Lancaster (p. 522) during his superintendency in the 1840s before becoming a Commissioner in Lunacy. This article also mentioned some of the other asylums in England, including the one at Wakefield, noting that "Samuel Tuke, explained instructions for the building of the Wakefield Pauper Lunatic Asylum" (p. 519) and that "Sir William Ellis, a wise and kindly man, ... first at Wakefield and afterwards at Hanwell, made the experiment of introducing labour systematically into our public asylums" (p. 521).

Wakefield does not appear to have been on the itinerary of Dickens's 1857 tour, although there was a visit to Doncaster, only about 20 miles distant. Hence it was not until after Dickens's death that the West Riding Asylum at Wakefield (henceforward WRA) was to feature in the pages of a Dickensian journal, *All the year round*.[5] Or, one should say, probably featured, since the article in question was anonymised. Nevertheless, a number of points in the article permit a definite identification to be made.

The "mad-doctor" named "Horniblow" who was the subject of the article is described as "the medical director of a large county asylum in the North of England" (p. 469), and as "a handsome, slightly-built man, with very fair hair, long blonde whiskers, the pleasantest of smiles, and the blandest and most conciliating manner" (p. 470). At the time of publication, September 1873, the medical superintendent at WRA was James Crichton-Browne (1840–1938), then in his early thirties, whose appearance was notable for his Dundreary whiskers. He had been appointed at WRA in 1866, and in recent years had developed the profile of the Asylum by setting up a dedicated pathological laboratory and photographic studio to permit the study of the brain in the hope of understanding the causes of insanity and developing treatments for its amelioration.[6]

Horniblow shares some anecdotes of asylum life with his visitor, for example one relating to a violent incident:

> Last March, one of our attendants, a strong active man, was watching an epileptic patient, and after poking the fire, he forgot to lock up the poker as he had been especially ordered to do. He had turned his back from the man and was looking out of the window at the patients exercising in the airing-court below. All at once the homicidal impulse came with the opportunity; the assassin stole softly behind him and killed him with one blow; after that beating the head to pieces (p. 470).

On 24th March 1871, one of the attendants at WRA, Thomas Lomas, had been killed in a similar manner when attacked by a patient, George Lawton. Crichton-Browne included the following account in his *Annual Report* to the Committee of Visitors for the year:

> a lamentable catastrophe involving the life of an attendant occurred on the 24th of March. The circumstances connected with the murder of Thomas Lomas, an able and experienced Attendant, by George Lawton, an epileptic patient, were at the time investigated by your Committee, so that it would be useless to repeat them now. The decision at which you arrived was, that no blame in connexion with the terrible event could be ascribed to any one, except the unfortunate man Lomas himself, who had neglected to lock away the poker after using it, as he had been specially instructed to do. Secure in his own strength and activity, he stood looking out at the window at his charges exercising in the airing court below, when his assassin with no grudge or animosity, but stirred by a pure homicidal impulse, an analogue of epilepsy convulsing the mind instead of the muscles, stole behind him, and dealt a blow, which was fatal in itself, but which was followed by others that reduced the head to a shapeless pulp.[7]

Accounts of the murder also appeared in the popular press.[8]

The visitor then asks Horniblow "Is it not injurious to patients to see visitors at these weekly dances that you give? Does it not excite them?" to which the director replies, speaking of "plays and dances" (p. 470). There was a tradition of amateur theatrical productions at WRA, introduced by Crichton-Browne, and following the innovation of his father, William A. F.

Browne (1805–1885), also a noted "mad-doctor," who inaugurated private theatricals when he was Superintendent at the Crichton Royal Institution in Dumfries (where James grew up) in 1843.[9] Members of the medical staff often took parts in the productions at WRA, sometimes parodying their own characters.

Horniblow then introduces his visitor to some of the asylum patients, one of whom is noted to be improving under treatment with the "Calabar bean" (p. 474). This was certainly one of the remedies used by Crichton-Browne. For example, writing in the WRA house journal, the *West Riding Lunatic Asylum Medical Reports* (henceforward *WRLAMR*), founded and edited by Crichton-Browne, one of the junior doctors at the Asylum, George Thompson, noted of the Calabar bean that "This drug has been used extensively by Dr. Crichton Browne, in the treatment of general paralysis in this asylum, and has been recommended by him as a valuable means of exercising a favourable influence on the course of the disease". Furthermore, "I do not exaggerate when I say that in every case very marked improvement has followed the use of the drug".[10]

These points are all suggestive, but more conclusive evidence that "Horniblow" and Crichton-Browne are one and the same is forthcoming. The visitor observes (p. 472) that "We certainly owe much to Gall and the phrenologists for drawing attention to the study of the brain, and for trying, however imperfectly, to localise the faculties" (Note that Finn, 2012:1, wrongly ascribed this statement to Horniblow). Horniblow replies that

"Doctor Browne, of the Crichton Royal Institution, has written a most curious and interesting essay on aphasia, or loss of speech in cerebral diseases, which bears on this subject; the doctor shows that it is certain some part of the brain must be injured before this loss arises, but then there are many sorts of deprivation. Doctor Browne gives some most extraordinary instances of this" (p. 472).

This "Doctor Browne" was none other than Crichton-Browne's father, Willam Browne. He had contributed a paper on aphasia to the 1872 volume of *WRLAMR*,[11] which included mention of patients "in this hospital" or explicitly "in the West Riding Asylum".

Horniblow then gives his visitor an example of a clinical phenomenon known as jargon aphasia:

"A patient at the West Riding Asylum, in 1868, uttered words all framed on this model. The following were words taken down from her lips, and all of them had a vague resemblance to Greek: 'Kallulios, tallulios, kaskos, tellulios, karoka, keka, tarrorei, kareka, sallullios'" (p. 473).

The identical jargon is also to be found in William Browne's paper in *WRLAMR*: "A characteristic exemplification of this symptom is afforded by the following passage, taken down from the lips of a patient in the West Riding Asylum, 3rd December, 1868".[11] The passage is also to be found in Crichton-Browne's musings published over 50 years later, although the two transcriptions are not identical. The retrospective account is as follows:

> "One of my medical assistants came and informed me that there was a female patient who was speaking Greek. On visiting her I found that she was repeating, in a loud, monotonous voice at the rate of ten times a minute, this piece of jargon of that alliterative type which jargon so often assumes:
>
> 'Kallulias, tallulios, Karekos,
> Tellulios, Karoka, Kareka,
> Karrorukareka, Salulios'".[12]

Since the jargon episode recounted by Horniblow to his visitor clearly had its origin at WRA and was witnessed and transcribed by Crichton-Browne, there can be no doubt about the identity of Horniblow and Crichton-Browne.

The *All the year round* article about Horniblow has certainly been accepted as referring to Crichton-Browne and WRA by later scholars: it forms the starting point for Michael Finn's thesis on the work at the Asylum during his superintendency[13] and was also noted by Neve and Turner in their paper on Crichton-Browne.[14] Finn noted some of the overlaps between the fictitious description and the factual record, but not the repetition of the jargon passage, nor the suggestive mention of the therapeutic use of Calabar bean.

The author of the article in *All the Year Round* is uncertain. It has been reported that "Records housed in the asylum museum indicate that Charles (Charley) Dickens (1837–96), the son of the novelist, visited the asylum in 1871, ... His interest seems to have been to provide copy for *All the Year Round*, of which he had become editor after his father's death the previous year".[15] If so, then the delay between a visit in 1871 and publication in September 1873 is difficult to explain. Certainly the profile of Crichton-Browne and WRA had risen in the intervening period, principally because of the experimental work undertaken in the Asylum laboratory by David Ferrier (1843–1928) in the Spring of 1873 which had gone some way "to localise the faculties" of the brain and which drew widespread attention in both medical and lay press.[16] Moreover, a visit in 1871 would predate William Browne's article in *WRLAMR*, although not the reported date of transcription of the jargon.

Acknowledgement

Unpublished manuscript, 5th August 2024.

References

1. Hilton C. 'A curious dance round a curious tree': Charles Dickens' visit to a mental hospital, Christmas 1851 (rcpsych.ac.uk) (Accessed 05/08/2024).
2. Williamson P. From confinement to community: the story of "The Moor", Lancaster's County Lunatic Asylum. In: S Wilson (ed.), *Aspects of Lancaster. Discovering local history.* Barnsley: Wharncliffe Books, 2002, p. 128.
3. The star of Bethlehem. *Household words* 1857; 16 (386): 145–150 (16th August).
4. Things within Dr. Conolly's remembrance. *Household words* 1857; 16 (401): 518–523 (28th November).
5. My friend the mad-doctor. *All the year round* 1873; 10 (250): 469–476 (13th September).
6. Todd J, Ashworth L. The West Riding Asylum and James Crichton-Browne, 1818–76. In: Berrios GE, Freeman H (eds.) *150 years of British Psychiatry 1841–1991.* London: Royal College of Psychiatrists, 1991, pp. 389–418.
7. *Report of the Committee of Visitors and of the Medical Superintendent of the West Riding Pauper Lunatic Asylum for the year 1871.* Wakefield: B.W. Allen, 1872, pp. 22–23.
8. Scrimgeour D. *Proper people. Early asylum life in the words of those who were there.* York: York Publishing, 2015, pp. 341–350.
9. Golding R. West Riding Asylum: Music and theatre in the large-scale pauper asylum. In: *Music and moral management in the Nineteenth-Century English lunatic asylum.* Cham: Palgrave Macmillan, 2021, pp. 129–156.
10. Thompson G. The sphygmograph in lunatic asylum practice. *West Riding Lunatic Asylum Medical Reports* 1871; 1: 58–70 [at 67, 70].
11. Browne WAF. Impairment of language, the result of cerebral disease. *West Riding Lunatic Asylum Medical Reports* 1872; 2: 278–301 [at 282; 284, 293, 299].
12. Crichton-Browne J. *Victorian jottings from an old commonplace book.* London: Etchells and Macdonald, 1926, pp. 59–60.
13. Finn MA. *The West Riding Lunatic Asylum and the making of the modern brain sciences in the nineteenth century.* Unpublished PhD thesis, University of Leeds, 2012. https://etheses.whiterose.ac.uk/3412/ (Accessed 05/08/24) [at 1–2].
14. Neve M, Turner T. What the Doctor thought and did: Sir James Crichton-Browne (1840–1938). *Med Hist* 1995; 39: 399–432 [at 406].
15. Wood J. A culture of improvement: knowledge, aesthetic consciousness, and the conversazione. *Nineteenth Century Studies* 2006 20: 79–97 [at 96n34].
16. Larner AJ. A month in the country: the sesquicentenary of David Ferrier's classical cerebral localisation researches of 1873. *Journal of the Royal College of Physicians of Edinburgh* 2023; 53: 128–131.

David Ferrier (1843–1928): *annus mirabilis* 1873

The *British Medical Journal* issue dated 26th April 1873 contained a "Preliminary Notice" contributed by David Ferrier, M.D., entitled "Experimental researches in cerebral physiology and pathology".[1] A medical graduate of Edinburgh University in 1868, Ferrier's current affiliations were listed as "Professor of Forensic Medicine in King's College; Junior Physician to the West London Hospital". However, the researches described had taken place far from the capital, in the West Yorkshire town of Wakefield, about 160 miles north of London. The paper began:

> The opportunity kindly afforded me by Dr Crichton Browne [*sic*], of experimenting on over thirty guinea-pigs, rabbits, cats, and dogs, in the pathological laboratory of the West Riding Asylum, Wakefield, has enabled me to arrive at certain results and conclusions which seem worthy of a brief preliminary notice, pending the publication of details of method, experiments, and illustrations, in the West Riding Asylum Reports [*sic*].

This modest paper, listing twelve "important conclusions" and taking up less than a column of print, summarised experimental findings which established the principle of cerebral localisation as physiological fact rather than, as previously, phrenological speculation. (These conclusions were also published in the October 1873 issue of the *Journal of Mental Science*.[2]) Ferrier (1843–1928) had undertaken the experiments to test the views of John Hughlings Jackson (1835–1911) on the pathology of epilepsy as a discharging lesion. James Crichton-Browne (1840–1938), the medical superintendent of the West Riding Pauper Lunatic Asylum in Wakefield from 1866 (and also an Edinburgh graduate, 1862), had established and equipped a pathological laboratory there in the year prior to Ferrier's arrival.

The preliminary report of Ferrier's findings was supplemented later in the year by the promised substantive paper, bearing the same title, which appeared in the *West Riding Lunatic Asylum Medical Reports* [henceforward *WRLAMR*],[3] the house journal of the West Riding Asylum which was edited by Crichton-Browne. This second paper may have appeared in July (elsewhere, Ferrier stated it appeared "in the beginning of August"[4]) and certainly by September (the volume of *WRLAMR* was reviewed in the issue of the *Medical Press and Circular* published on 3rd September[5]). The paper mentioned experiments on pigeons and fowls, in addition to guinea-pigs, rabbits, cats, and dogs. Furthermore, in a footnote in this paper (Ref. 3, p.89n2), Ferrier reported that "I have now (June 14) ascertained the position of all these centres in the brain of the monkey, and therefore, by implication, their situation in man. These experiments will soon be published".

The monkey studies were undertaken in London with funding from the Royal Society. (Exactly where these studies were performed is, to my knowledge, unstated. Possibilities include the Brown Animal Sanatory Institution in Lambeth, with which Ferrier had previously been associated; or King's College London, where Ferrier's later collaborative animal research took place in the Physiological Laboratory.) This extended experimental work – "I operated on nearly a hundred animals of all classes – fish, frogs, fowls, pigeons, rats, guinea pigs, rabbits, cats, dogs, jackalls [*sic*], and monkeys" – was mentioned in a note published in *Nature* on 2nd October 1873.[5] The monkey work was also referred to in a brief paper in the *Journal of Anatomy and Physiology* dated November 1873,[6] (but, according to Samuel Greenblatt,[7] "published in 1874"; p.514) prior to the definitive publications in the house journals of the Royal Society in 1874 and 1875.[8-11] (NB I take the dating of Experiment XIV in Ref. 11, p.459, printed as "March 9th, 1873", to be a typographical error for 1875, since the latter fits with the sequence of Experiments XII, XIII, and XV. As will be shown, Ferrier may already have been in Wakefield on this date.)

How had it come about that Ferrier journeyed to Wakefield to initiate these researches rather than pursue them at King's College? I am not aware of any direct contemporary sources, but according to Charles Scott Sherrington (1857–1952) writing in 1928:

> In March 1873, when he [Ferrier] was paying a visit to his friend and fellow Edinburgh graduate, Dr. (now Sir) James Crichton-Browne, then Director of the West Riding Asylum, Wakefield, conversation turned upon the excitability under galvanism of part of the cerebral surface of the dog as reported from the Continent by Fritsch and Hitzig [1870]. There followed, during the course of the spring and summer of 1873, in the laboratory recently founded at the Asylum ... the memorable experiments with which Ferrier opened his detailed systematic exploration by faradic stimulation of all parts of the central nervous system in representative types of vertebrate from the lowest to the highest.[12]

This account was written for Ferrier's obituary, hence more than 50 years after the events described. Some caution as to its accuracy may therefore be appropriate, even accepting that Ferrier and Sherrington were friends (Sherrington's magnum opus *The Integrative Action of the Nervous System* of 1906 was dedicated to Ferrier).

Other, much later, sources place Ferrier's conversation with Crichton-

Browne at different times. We may safely discount Edwin Clarke's dating (his account is otherwise largely taken from Sherrington's):

> ... early in 1878 [*sic*] Ferrier discussed it [the work of Fritsch & Hitzig, 1870] with his friend and fellow student at Edinburgh, Sir James Crichton-Browne, director of the West Riding Lunatic Asylum at Wakefield. As a result, during the spring and summer of that year Ferrier carried out investigations in the laboratory recently installed at the asylum.[13]

Although Ferrier and Crichton-Browne both studied at Edinburgh, they were not contemporaries; Crichton-Browne left in 1862, and Ferrier did not arrive until 1865. However, they were certainly both influenced by the teaching of Thomas Laycock, Chair of the Practice of Physic at Edinburgh University from 1855, who had initiated instruction in medical psychology and mental diseases.

Michael Finn's gives an earlier date, but without reference(s):

> Late in 1872, when Crichton-Browne's good friend and fellow Scotsman Ferrier visited Wakefield for the annual conversazione, the two talked about many things, and Fritsch and Hitzig's results were chief among them. ... Crichton-Browne ... thus invited Ferrier back in March to conduct more electrical experiments in rooms of the asylum.[14]

The annual meetings, termed *conversazione*, were another innovation introduced by Crichton-Browne at the West Riding Asylum. Occurring between 1871 and 1875, the *conversazione* certainly attracted "men of science" as well as local practitioners, but the five-line report of the meeting of 15th October 1872 published in the *Lancet* (1872;2:615) mentions no names other than that of the keynote speaker, Professor William Turner of Edinburgh, who lectured on the cerebral convolutions (he was also a co-founder and editor of the *Journal of Anatomy and Physiology*). A "List of the gentlemen invited" printed in the *Leeds Mercury* newspaper of 17th October 1872 (p.8. Medical Conversazione at the West Riding Asylum) does not include Ferrier's name.

However, one contemporary record does provide some additional information. In a letter to Charles Darwin (1809–1882) dated 16th April 1873, Crichton-Browne states:

> Professor Ferrier of King's College *has just completed* an experimental investigation in my pathological laboratory which cannot fail to interest you and which must have an incalculable bearing on your views. By exposing the brains of living animals, under chloroform, and stimulating the cerebral grey matter by an electric current from Du Bois Reymond's

[induction] coil he has discovered that every convolution of the brain is in direct relation with certain groups of muscles, and controls their actions. ... Professor Ferrier's researches which are to be published in the next volume of West Riding Asylum Medical Reports [*sic*] in July, will I believe constitute the most important advances yet made in cerebral physiology [my italics].[15]

This dating would seem to discount the report of Milner Fothergill, a friend of Ferrier's in London, who also published in *WRLAMR*, who mentioned in passing in a paper published the following year that "Dr. Ferrier's experiments ... commenced at Wakefield Asylum last Easter".[16] Easter Sunday fell on the 13th April in 1873.

These contemporary accounts also invalidate Crichton-Browne's recollections published over 50 years later (1926) to the effect that:

Professor Turner (afterwards Sir William Turner) was spending three days with us in October 1872, and delivered a very important and suggestive address at our medical conversazione on "The Convolutions of the Human Brain in relation to the Intelligence". Reviewing Ferrier's recent observations in my laboratory on the localisation of function in the brain, he said ... [17]

As noted, William Turner lectured at WRA on 15th October 1872, but this predated Ferrier's experimental observations on localisation by around 6 months. Crichton-Browne might perhaps have become confused because the publication of Turner's lecture and of Ferrier's experimental findings appeared as consecutive papers in the third volume of *WRLAMR*. Moreover, Turner's printed text of 1873 included mention in a footnote of the abstract of Ferrier's results published in April 1873 in the *BMJ*[1] and awareness but not sight of his substantive *WRLAMR* paper.[3] Turner, as co-editor of the *Journal of Anatomy and Physiology*, may have been instrumental in Ferrier's subsequent publication in that journal.[6]

Thus, if Ferrier arrived in Wakefield to begin his work in March 1873, as per Sherrington's account,[12] and had completed it by mid April, as per Crichton-Browne's letter to Darwin,[15] it would seem that in little over a month he had made his key observations and was ready to go into print. The site of his experimental work now shifted back to London for the monkey experiments; *contra* Sherrington, it does not seem that Ferrier undertook any further experimental work at Wakefield in the summer of 1873, or indeed at any future date. He did avail himself of the Asylum's written resources for a second *WRLAMR* paper (*vide infra*), and this may have been at a later date.

As noted by Sherrington,[12] one of the principal stimuli to Ferrier's experimental studies, in addition to Hughlings Jackson's clinical inferences, was the work of Gustav Fritsch (1838–1927) and Eduard Hitzig (1838–1907) who in 1870 had reported localised centres for various movements in response to galvanic stimulation in the cortex of the dog.[18] Certainly Ferrier had been aware of this work since at least the early months of 1871, as it was one of the papers reviewed in a publication which he had co-authored.[19] As he had travelled to Heidelberg in 1864, apparently visiting the laboratories of Hermann von Helmholtz and Wilhelm Wundt (although this may be a later assumption), he had a working knowledge of German and so was well able to comprehend and assimilate these new findings. Ferrier certainly mentioned the work of Fritsch and Hitzig in his 1873 papers (e.g. in the second conclusion of his *BMJ* paper[1]) but evidently felt that he had gone beyond them, both in method (faradic rather than galvanic stimulation) and extent (species examined, centres identified). Hitzig, however, was vocal in his feelings about under (rather than lack of) acknowledgement, sentiments shared by the referees of Ferrier's initial report to the Royal Society[20] and the author(s) of an (anonymous) editorial in *Nature*.[21] Young has suggested that thereafter Ferrier's references to Fritsch and Hitzig were more generous,[20] although it cannot be doubted that Ferrier advanced the field far beyond their initial study.

Awareness of, and response to, Ferrier's researches was prompt. On 10th May 1873, just two weeks after the initial report, Hughlings Jackson responded in the *British Medical Journal*.[22]

Greenblatt, in his biography of Hughlings Jackson,[7] states in his discussion of this paper that it shows Jackson clearly had prior knowledge of Ferrier's primate results suggesting that the two men were in contact at this time (pp. 166–168).

Further comment from Hughlings Jackson appeared in the 12th July issue of the *Medical Times and Gazette*.[23] Writing on "A series of cases illustrative of cerebral pathology: cases of intra-cranial tumour", Hughlings Jackson noted that "Such cases have their interest much widened by the recent researches of Dr. Ferrier: the artificial production of convulsions by galvanising the convolutions. (a)". [Ferrier had in fact used faradic stimulation, unlike Fritsch and Hitzig who used galvanic stimulation.] The footnote, (a), stated that "Dr. Ferrier has given a very brief statement of his main results in the Brit. Med. J., April 26, 1873. A full account of his researches will appear in the forthcoming volume of Dr Crichton Browne's West Riding Asylum Reports. ... I have already briefly remarked on this elsewhere (Brit. Med. J., May 10), and shall do so more fully in the next volume of Crichton Browne's reports" (p. 33 and n(a)). I presume this refers to Jackson's paper entitled "Observations on localisation of movements in the cerebral hemispheres, as revealed by cases of convulsion, chorea and 'aphasia'" which appeared in the third volume of

WRLAMR (pp. 175–195). Certainly this paper[24] begins with an with acknowledgement of Ferrier's work as confirming Jackson's view that discharges of convolutions develop movements, referring to Ferrier's *BMJ* paper.[1] Likewise Jackson's second paper in the same volume of *WRLAMR* (pp. 315–349) which reproduces the 4th and 5th conclusions from Ferrier's *BMJ* paper (p. 317n1).[25] According to Greenblatt (p.174n84),[7] Jackson's first reference to Ferrier's substantive *WRLAMR* paper[3] was in a publication in the *Lancet* dated 13th December 1873.[26]

Ferrier's work was also mentioned and/or discussed in several addresses published in the *British Medical Journal* in 1873, some delivered at the 41st Annual Meeting of the British Medical Association held in London in early August of that year. For example, Harrington Tuke stated that "Dr Ferrier is at this moment engaged in a series of scientific experiments, bearing on the nature and treatment of insanity ... at the West Riding Asylum" (*BMJ* 1873;2:189; 16th Aug issue; also reported in *J Ment Sci* 1873–1874;19:486; October 1873 issue). John Burdon Sanderson (1828–1905), the editor of the *Handbook for the physiological laboratory* published in 1873, which described many physiological animal experiments but controversially without mention of anaesthesia, and with whom Ferrier had previously worked in London, discussed "the very extended and laborious experimental investigation of the motor functions of the brain, of which some of us have seen the results" (*BMJ* 1873;2:197; 16th Aug issue).

For those not privy to those results, the opportunity was available to see a demonstration of the findings for themselves, since on 8th August (the same day as Burdon Sanderson's address):

> Dr FERRIER experimented upon a cat and a monkey. After removing the vault of the cranium and the dura mater, he faradised various portions of the convolutions in succession. In applying his electrodes to the several convolutions, Dr Ferrier predicted movements, for example, of the foot, the shoulder, the ear, the mouth, the eye, the head, etc.; and almost always the predicted movement occurred. ... We believe that the researches of which Dr Ferrier gave examples are regarded by competent physiologists as of very great importance (*BMJ* 1873;2:241).

Ferrier's work was also discussed in the *Medical Times and Gazette* issue of 30th August, which reproduced the twelve conclusions from his initial *BMJ* paper, and stated that "His researches are published in the current (third) volume of the 'West Riding Lunatic Asylum Report [*sic*]'",[27] indicating that this volume was published by this time (and corroborating Ferrier's later comment concerning the timing of publication[4]). The *WRLAMR* paper was also commented on in the *Dublin Journal of Medical Science*.[28]

Ferrier had a further opportunity to disseminate his findings in September 1873, at the 43rd Annual Meeting of the British Association for the Advancement of Science held in Bradford, West Yorkshire. His address, entitled "On the Localisation of the functions of the brain," was presented on Friday 19th September and this formed the substance of his note published in *Nature* the following month.[5] The presentation was reported in the 27th September issue of the *Lancet* (1873;2:459) which noted that part of these researches had already appeared in the "Medical Reports of the West Riding Lunatic Asylum [*sic*]", but although Ferrier's monkey data were not to hand nevertheless "Such physiological researches as these proceeding from an English laboratory present an exceedingly satisfactory sign of the times and will, we hope, be the prelude to many others of equal value". According to the correspondent in the 4th October issue of the *Lancet*, this was "the most important communication made in the Section of Biology during the meeting. The large room was positively crammed during its delivery, which occupied nearly two hours" (*Lancet* 1873;2:503–504). The brief report in the *Medical Press and Circular* of 24th September (1873;16:275) hailed an "entirely new system of phrenology". Comment also appeared in the *Medical Times and Gazette* of 27th September (1873;2:357–8), as well as a report of Ferrier's presentation and the following discussion,[29] and also in the *Boston Medical and Surgical Journal* (1873;88:419). Also appearing on 27th September, the report in *The Examiner* (1873;Issue 3426:966–967) noted, perhaps unhelpfully, Ferrier's method as "a new mode of interrogating nature – a new instrument of torture, so to speak, by which more of her secrets could be extracted", although the use of chloroform in all experiments was stated.

At the West Riding Asylum *conversazione* of 25th November 1873, William Carpenter was the keynote speaker, his presentation entitled "On the physiological import of Dr Ferrier's experimental investigations into the functions of the brain". This was undoubtedly one of the two lectures alluded to in the *British Medical Journal* (1873;2:641; 29th Nov issue) as recently given by Carpenter on the functions of the brain, and Ferrier was listed as one of those present (*Lancet* 1873;2:788; 29th Nov issue). Indeed, the programme for the *conversazione* (reproduced by Spillane[30]) reports that "During the course of the evening, David Ferrier … will demonstrate 'The localisation of function in the brain'". Aminoff, citing Spillane, says that Ferrier "lectured",[31] but from the accounts in the contemporary popular press it is quite clear that Ferrier undertook experimental demonstrations, as at the British Medical Association meeting in London in August. The *Leeds Mercury* newspaper of 27th November 1873 (p.7) stated that "A series of experiments were … made by Dr. Ferrier upon a cat under chloroform in demonstration of the localisation of function in the brain" (cited by Crowther[32]). However, a much fuller account appeared in the *Yorkshire Post and Leeds Intelligencer* of the same date (p.3). After Carpenter's talk:

> a most interesting part of the business of the evening took place. In a small room off the hall, Professor Ferrier gave to parties of 12 or 14 gentlemen at a time, demonstrations of "The Localisation of Function in the Brain." The experiments were made upon a cat, which having been placed under chloroform, the covering of the brain was removed. The interest and importance of the experiments consisted in the definiteness and certainty with which certain muscular movements were produced, on the application of the electrode to certain portions of the brain. ... The interest evinced in the experiments was very great, there being quite a rush of gentlemen to witness them. ... The company did not separate until a late hour.

The Wakefield Express, and Barnsley, Normanton, Pontefract, Ossett, Horbury & Dewsbury Advertiser (Vol. 22, No. 1126, 29th November 1873, p.2, cols. 6–7) noted that Ferrier "applied the electrodes of a galvanic battery ... first testing the strength of the current ... by applying them to his own tongue, and predicting the movements which would ensue" and that "When the experiments were completed the animal was destroyed...".

As the audience consisted of nearly 300 medical men one can understand why the meeting ran late if all or even most were witnesses of Ferrier's demonstration.

In the same issue of the *Lancet* which reported the 1873 West Riding Asylum *conversazione*, a note informed readers that:

> Dr Ferrier has received a grant from the Royal Society for the purpose of enabling him to pursue his investigations upon the brains of monkeys, &c. The results of his experiments will in due time be embodied in a paper which he will read before the Society (*Lancet* 1873;2:788).

Although monkey studies had been in progress at least since June 1873,[3] were publicly demonstrated in August, and adverted to in a presentation in September and a publication in October,[5] the substantive papers on this aspect of Ferrier's work did not appear until 1874–1875,[8-11] followed in 1876 by the monograph *The functions of the brain* (second edition 1886).[33]

At the end of 1873, in its 27th December issue, the *BMJ* published a report of "Ferrier's experimental researches in cerebral physiology and pathology" based on his publications of that year.[34] Also in December, the retiring President of the Royal Society, Sir George Airy, noted in his address reviewing the year that "In Anatomy [*sic*], the most striking subject appears to be Professor

Ferrier's experimental discussion of the actions of different parts of the brain, explained at the late Meeting of the British Association".[35]

Evidently Ferrier's work had also gained an international dimension by the end of 1873. In the USA, the *Boston Medical and Surgical Journal* (forerunner of the *New England Journal of Medicine*) mentioned Ferrier's initial *BMJ* paper in two separate reports (one, by Henry Pickering Bowditch, misdated the paper as 26th April 1872).[36,37] The *Chicago Journal of Nervous and Mental Disease* (forerunner of the *Journal of Nervous and Mental Disease*) only commenced publication in January 1874 but its very first issue noted Ferrier's work,[38] reprinting his *Journal of Anatomy and Physiology paper*[6] in its entirety. By this time, the experimental techniques had been taken up by more investigators and in other countries, including Roberts Bartholow's infamous experiment upon his patient Mary Rafferty published in April 1874,[39,40] leading to some differences in interpretation of Ferrier's results.[41] In France, the first of 13 instalments translating Ferrier's *WRLAMR* paper appeared in *Le Progrès Médical* on 20 December 1873,[42] the remainder appearing in 1874, then collected as a pamphlet.

Ferrier's experiments had also excited wider public notice, not least within the anti-vivisection movement,[43] eventually leading to a Royal Commission under Lord Cardwell and thence to the passage of the Cruelty to Animals Act 1876, under the terms of which Ferrier was later (1881) unsuccessfully prosecuted.[44] However, it seems that Ferrier was alive to potential criticisms of his work from the anti-vivisectionists much earlier, since in the 1873 substantive paper[3] he noted that the animals had to be experimented upon under the influence of chloroform or ether "not only from humane motives, but to exclude the complication of voluntary or reflex movements" (p.33) and also stated "once for all, that before and throughout all the following experiments, ether or chloroform was administered" (p.35). This may be an early example of what Boddice has termed the editorial self-consciousness of medical scientists with respect to vivisection following the publication of Burdon Sanderson's *Handbook for the physiological laboratory* and the controversy surrounding its omission of details of anaesthesia.[45]

From the outset, Ferrier was considering the implications of his findings not only for the physiology of motor function and the pathology of cerebral disease such as epileptic seizures but also for higher mental functions. In his first paper, conclusion number 1 stated: "The anterior portions of the cerebral hemisphere are the chief centres of voluntary motion and the active outward manifestation of intelligence".[1] In the second, substantive paper, he questioned whether "ideational centres" were situated in the same regions as the corresponding motor centres, and in favour of this possibility cited the "now tolerably well established fact of loss of speech following destructive lesions of the lower frontal convolutions in the neighbourhood of the Island of Reil".[3] Aphasia was thus conceptualised as destruction of the centres of word memory: "The part of the brain which is the seat of the memory of words is that which governs the movements of the mouth and the tongue".[5] Hence in Ferrier's view "The pathology of aphasia is thus rendered comparatively simple" because the patient is unable to "lay hold of the word which he wishes to express".[6]

More on the ramifications of Ferrier's findings for "psychical manifestations" (what we might now term cognitive and behavioural symptoms) was to follow. In a second *West Riding Lunatic Asylum Medical Reports* paper, published in 1874, Ferrier attempted clinico-pathological correlation in five patients, based on their details as recorded in the West Riding Asylum casebooks, in order "to show the clinical bearings of experimental researches on the functions of the brain".[46] (My speculation is that Ferrier took the opportunity of his visit to the Asylum to present at the conversazione in November 1873 to examine the case books and post-mortem books.) These five patients had diagnoses of epileptic insanity, epileptic mania (both with defects of memory), dementia, aphasia, and melancholia. Perhaps the clearest correlation was in the aphasic patient: loss of speech output for all but single syllable words beginning with "b" yet preserved language comprehension, accompanied by right hemiplegia and dementia, in association with a destructive lesion of the left hemisphere. Perhaps the least clear correlation was in the melancholic: the "symptoms not altogether easy of explanation by the lesions of the brain discovered on post-mortem examination". Ferrier's conclusion was prescient: "though much yet requires to be done, especially in reference to the psychical function of the brain, there is every reason to believe that the union of physiological experimentation with pathological observation will ultimately succeed in unravelling even this obscure subject, and establishing mental physiology and pathology on a more tangible basis".[46]

It should be noted that these conclusions predated the evolution of the neurological examination as we know it. At this time, neurological examination was still in a rudimentary state – even the knee jerk was not described until the following year (by Erb and by Westphal),[47,48] let alone evaluation of cognitive and behavioural symptoms. Hence Ferrier's distrust of inferences drawn from clinical as opposed to experimental material was no doubt well justified, as expressed in his monograph on *The functions of the brain* (1876:xiv):

> ... experiments on animals, under conditions selected and varied at the will of the experimenter, are alone capable of furnishing precise data for sound inductions as to the functions of the brain and its various parts; the

experiments performed for us by nature, in the form of diseased conditions, being rarely limited, or free from such complications as render analysis and the discovery of cause and effect extremely difficult, and in many cases practically impossible.

As shown in the foregoing account, which does not claim to be exhaustive, all Ferrier's key observations were made and reported in 1873 and were already widely disseminated and commented upon by the end of that year. Hence, it was appropriate to commemorate, and celebrate, 2023 as the sesquicentenary of Ferrier's pioneering work on cerebral localisation.

Acknowledgement

Adapted and greatly extended from: Larner AJ. A month in the country: the sesquicentenary of David Ferrier's classical cerebral localisation researches of 1873. *J R Coll Physicians Edinb* 2023;53:128–131. The title of this paper was based on the play of Ivan Turgenev (first staged 1872) and the novel of JL Carr (1980; film 1987).

References

1. Ferrier D. Experimental researches in cerebral physiology and pathology. *Br Med J* 1873; 1: 457.
2. Anon. *J Ment Sci* 1873–1874; 19 (October 1873): 468–9.
3. Ferrier D. Experimental researches in cerebral physiology and pathology. *West Riding Lunatic Asylum Medical Reports* 1873; 3: 30–96. [Available online at: https://archive.org/details/39002086346286.med.yale.edu/page/30/mode/2up]
4. Ferrier D. Hitzig on experiments on the brain. *London Medical Record* 1874; 2: 399–402 [at 399].
5. Ferrier [D]. The localisation of the functions in the brain. *Nature* 1873; 8: 477–8.
6. Ferrier D. Experimental researches in cerebral physiology and pathology. *J Anat Physiol* 1873; 8: 152–5.
7. Greenblatt SH. *John Hughlings Jackson. Clinical neurology, evolution, and Victorian brain science.* Oxford: Oxford University Press, 2022.
8. Ferrier D. The localization [*sic*] of function in the brain (Abstract). *Proc R Soc Lond* 1874; 22: 229–32.
9. Ferrier D. Experiments on the brain of monkeys – No. 1. *Proc R Soc Lond* 1874; 23: 409–30.
10. Ferrier D. The Croonian Lecture, "Experiments on the brain of monkeys" (Second Series). *Proc R Soc Lond* 1875; 23: 431–2.
11. Ferrier D. The Croonian Lecture. Experiments on the brain of monkeys (Second Series). *Phil Trans R Soc Lond* 1875; 165: 433–88.

12. Sherrington CS. Sir David Ferrier, 1843–1928. *Proc R Soc Lond B Biol Sci* 1928; 103: viii-xvi.
13. Clarke E. https://www.encyclopedia.com/science/dictionaries-thesauruses-pictures-and-press-releases/ferrier-david (accessed 09/05/23).
14. Finn MA. *The West Riding Lunatic Asylum and the making of the modern brain sciences in the nineteenth century.* Unpublished PhD thesis, University of Leeds, 2012, p.139. https://etheses.whiterose.ac.uk/3412/ (accessed 22/01/23).
15. Darwin Correspondence Project, "Letter no. 8861," https://www.darwinproject.ac.uk/letter/?docld=letters/DCP-LETT-8861.xml (accessed 22/01/23).
16. Fothergill JM. The depressants of the circulation and their use. *Br Med J* 1874; 1: 77–9 [at 77].
17. Crichton-Browne J. *Victorian jottings from an old commonplace book.* London: Etchells and Macdonald, 1926:111.
18. Fritsch G, Hitzig E. Über die elektrische Erregbarkeit des Grosshirns [On the electrical excitability of the cerebrum]. *Archiv für Anatomie, Physiologie und Wissenschaftliche Medicin* 1870; 37: 300–32. [Reprinted in *Epilepsy Behav* 2009; 15: 123–30.]
19. Fraser TR, Brunton TL, Ferrier D. Report on the progress of physiology: from 1st January to 1st April, 1871. *J Anat Physiol* 1871; 5(2): 389–411 [at 396].
20. Young RM. *Mind, brain and adaptation in the nineteenth century: cerebral localization and its biological context from Gall to Ferrier.* Oxford: Clarendon Press, 1970: 234–48.
21. Anon. Hitzig v. Ferrier. *Nature* 1874; 10: 259.
22. Jackson JH. On the anatomical investigation of epilepsy and epileptiform convulsions. *Br Med J* 1873; 1: 531–3.
23. Jackson JH. A series of cases illustrative of cerebral pathology: cases of intracranial tumour. *Medical Times and Gazette* 1873; 2: 33–5.
24. Jackson JH. Observations on the localisation of movements in the cerebral hemispheres, as revealed by cases of convulsion, chorea, and "aphasia". *West Riding Lunatic Asylum Medical Reports* 1873; 3: 175–95.
25. Jackson JH. On the anatomical, physiological, and pathological investigation of epilepsies. *West Riding Lunatic Asylum Medical Reports* 1873; 3: 315–49.
26. Jackson JH. London Hospital. Remarks on limited convulsive seizures, and on the after-effects of strong nervous discharges. *Lancet* 1873; 2: 840–1.
27. Anon. Researches in the physiology and pathology of the brain. *Medical Times and Gazette* 1873; 2: 233–4.
28. Anon. Investigations regarding cerebral pathology. *Dublin Journal of Medical Science* 1873; 56: 374–6.
29. Anon. Professor Ferrier on the localisation of functions in the brain. *Medical Times and Gazette* 1873; 2: 362–3.
30. Spillane JD. A memorable decade in the history of neurology 1874–84. I. *Br Med J* 1974; 4: 701–6 [Fig. 4 at p.704].
31. Aminoff MJ. *Victor Horsley. The world's first neurosurgeon and his conscience.*

Cambridge: Cambridge University Press, 2022, p.40.

32. Crowther A. *Pygmalion* at the Asylum. *W.S. Gilbert Society Journal* 2013; 5 (32): 5–21 [at 13 and n13].
33. Ferrier D. *The functions of the brain*. London: Smith, Elder & Co., 1876.
34. Anon. Ferrier's experimental researches in cerebral physiology and pathology. *Br Med J* 1873; 2: 767–8.
35. Airy GB. President's address. *Proc R Soc Lond* 1873–4; 22: 2–12 [at 9].
36. Bowditch HP. Report on physiology. *Boston Med Surg J* 1873; 88: 79–82 [at 80; Ferrier's original paper misdated as 26th April 1872 at 79].
37. Fisher TW. Report on mental diseases. *Boston Med Surg J* 1873; 88: 104–14 [at 107].
38. Anon. Recent progress in cerebral physiology. *J Nerv Ment Dis* 1874; 1: 52–9 [at 55–9; Ferrier's *J Anat Physiol* paper reprinted at 56–8].
39. Bartholow R. Experimental investigations into the functions of the human brain. *Am J Med Sci* 1874; 67: 305–13.
40. Harris LJ, Almerigi JB. Probing the human brain with stimulating electrodes: the story of Roberts Bartholow's (1874) experiment on Mary Rafferty. *Brain Cogn* 2009; 70: 92–115.
41. Ferrier D. On the localisation of the functions of the brain. *Br Med J* 1874; 2: 766–7.
42. Ferrier D (transl. Duret H). Recherches expérimentales sur la Physiologie et la Pathologie cérébrales. *Le Progrès Médical* 1873; 1(28): 333–4.
43. Finn MA, Stark JF. Medical science and the Cruelty to Animals Act 1876: a re-examination of anti-vivisectionism in provincial Britain. *Studies in History and Philosophy of Biological and Biomedical Sciences* 2015; 49: 12–23.
44. Bone I, Larner AJ. The trial of David Ferrier, November 1881: context, proceedings, and aftermath. *J Hist Neurosci* 2024; 33: 333–354.
45. Boddice R. *Humane professions: the defence of experimental medicine, 1876–1914*. Cambridge: Cambridge University Press, 2021: 159n61.
46. Ferrier D. Pathological illustrations of brain function. *West Riding Lunatic Asylum Medical Reports* 1874; 4: 30–62.
47. Lazar JW. The early history of the knee-jerk reflex in neurology. *J Hist Neurosci* 2022; 31: 409–24.
48. Adan G, Larner AJ. Sesquicentenary of the knee jerk reflex: the contributions of Hughlings Jackson, Horsley, and Sherrington. *J Hist Neurosci* (in press).

William Bevan-Lewis (1847–1929)

William Bevan-Lewis was a pioneer in the field of neuropathology in the late 19th and early 20th centuries who is best remembered for his discoveries in histological localisation of the cerebral cortex [1]. For 35 years he worked at the West Riding Lunatic Asylum at Wakefield in Yorkshire, United Kingdom, an institution wherein the scientific foundations of neurology received particular impetus from the 1870s onwards. Although he approached the subject from the perspective of an alienist or medical psychologist (what we would now term a psychiatrist or neuropsychiatrist), he was described by one of his successors as a neurologist [2], reflecting the porosity of these professional categories at the time.

Born in Cardigan in the west of Wales, he trained at Guy's Hospital in London, qualifying in 1868. He gained initial experience as an assistant medical officer at Buckingham County Asylum but, having married young, was obliged to pursue private practice in Cardigan which he found uncongenial. The key event in determining his career was his appointment as a Clinical Assistant (unpaid!) to the West Riding Asylum (WRA) in 1875 [3]. WRA was then (1866–1876) under the superintendency of James Crichton-Browne (1840–1938) and was an active research school with its own journal, the *West Riding Lunatic Asylum Medical Reports* (*WRLAMR*), wherein David Ferrier and John Hughlings Jackson had published seminal contributions on cerebral localisation based on animal experimentation and clinical observation (epileptic phenomena), respectively [4]. Bevan-Lewis published his first paper, "On the histology of the great sciatic nerve in general paralysis of the insane" in *WRLAMR* in 1875. Two further papers followed before *WRLAMR* ceased publication in 1876. He was then a prolific contributor to *Brain*, effectively the successor journal to *WRLAMR*, as well as publishing in *The Lancet*, *BMJ*, and the *Journal of Mental Science* (forerunner of the *British Journal of Psychiatry*). He also attended the WRA medical *conversazione* of 1875, manning a table with Herbert Major displaying microscopical preparations.

In 1878, Bevan-Lewis published with Henry Clarke a seminal paper on cerebral cytoarchitectonics, building on the work of Meynert, and illustrating for the first time the large pyramidal ("ganglionic") cells previously described by Betz and showing their distribution, thus localising the motor area anterior to the central sulcus of Rolando. The authors favoured a five-layered model of the motor area [5]. Bevan-Lewis's paper in the inaugural issue of *Brain* (April 1878) "On the comparative structure of the cortex cerebri" was an extension of this work and was followed by comparative studies in various animals (rat,

69

rabbit, pig, sheep, cat, ocelot, Barbary macaque), work supported by a government grant.

Lewis's hybrid model of cortical cytoarchitectonics was made clear here: "There is a five and a six-laminated cortex, each typical of a certain definite area: but, whilst the six-layered formation is found extensively spread over the convolutions of the parietal and other regions, the *five-laminated* type is pre-eminently characteristic of the motor area of the brain" [6]. He did not depart from this view in later publications.

A series of six papers on "Methods of preparing, demonstrating, and examining cerebral structure in health and disease" appeared in *Brain* between 1880 and 1882, and formed the subject matter of his first book, *The Human Brain. Histological and Coarse Methods of Research. A Manual for Students and Asylum Officers*, published in 1882 [7]. These various studies not only demonstrated his facility with microscopic techniques but also use of the freezing microtome to cut thin sections of brain tissue. His familiarity with various staining techniques was instrumental in his later description of "spider cells" (what we would now term astrocytes) in the cerebral cortex from patients with general paralysis of the insane [8]. He also made use of the photographic facilities established at WRA by Crichton-Browne to illustrate his works.

Bevan-Lewis's magnum opus, *A Text-book of Mental Diseases*, first appeared in 1889 (second edition 1899) and summarised his wealth of neuropathological and clinical experience, including observations on the deleterious effects of alcohol on the brain [8]. It was acknowledged to be "without doubt, the best English book of its kind" by the reviewer in the *Journal of Mental Science*. Bevan-Lewis also contributed the chapter on the pathology of the nervous system in the multi-volume *System of Medicine* edited by Clifford Allbutt, a physician who had worked at WRA in the 1860s and 1870s. Throughout his years at Wakefield Bevan-Lewis was also Lecturer and Examiner in Mental Diseases to the Yorkshire College [8], later the University of Leeds; this post became a professorship when the Leeds School of Medicine became a University Faculty.

Despite his focus on neuropathological research, Bevan-Lewis did not neglect the administrative duties incumbent upon mental asylum officers. He became Superintendent of WRA in 1884 and remained in post for 26 years, during which time he inaugurated an Outpatient Department (1889), reconstructed the Pathology Department to include a complete outfit of laboratories by 1895, and oversaw the planning and building of a new acute hospital on the site (opened in 1900). He also witnessed the founding of further branches of WRA, at Menston (1888) and Storthes Hall (1904). He supported many young researchers during his superintendency, ensuring that research did not cease to emerge from WRA. He was elected President of the Medico-Psychological

Association for 1909–1910 [9] prior to his retirement from WRA in 1910.

There is some inconsistency in the hyphenation of his name (as is the case for Hughlings Jackson and Crichton-Browne). The hyphen was present in his obituaries [2,3] (hence its adoption here), yet absent in his publications in the *West Riding Lunatic Asylum Medical Reports*, in *Brain* (where he published as "Dr Bevan Lewis"), and in the three editions of his two books [6,7]. However, the hyphen was present by the time of his address "On the Formation of Character" to the nursing staff at the York Retreat (November 1906) and in his presidential address to the Medico-Psychological Association (1909) [8].

Bevan-Lewis died at the age of 82 years in 1929. In his obituaries (all of which use the hyphenated surname [2,3,10]), he was described by Crichton-Browne as "one of the gentlest and most unobtrusive of men ... [who] persistently kept himself in the background" [3], and by Joseph Shaw Bolton as "an enthusiast, and a recluse with few interests beyond his scientific investigations" despite which he "justly acquired a great scientific reputation, and his position as a neurologist of the highest rank" [2]. His self-effacing character may be one reason why his work, although acknowledged in some recent publications [11,12], is not well-known to posterity.

Acknowledgement

Adapted from: Larner AJ, Triarhou LC. William Bevan-Lewis (1847–1929). *J Neurol* 2023;270:1190–1191.

References

1. Triarhou LC (2021) Pre-Brodmann pioneers of cortical cytoarchitectonics I: Theodor Meynert, Vladimir Betz and William Bevan-Lewis. Brain Struct Funct 226:49–67
2. Anonymous (1929) Obituary. William Bevan-Lewis, M.Sc. Leeds, M.R.C.S., L.S.A. Lancet 2:954–955
3. Anonymous (1929) William Bevan-Lewis, M.Sc., M.R.C.S. Br Med J 2:833–834
4. Finn MA (2012) The West Riding Lunatic Asylum and the making of the modern brain sciences in the nineteenth century. Unpublished PhD thesis, University of Leeds. https://etheses.whiterose.ac.uk/3412/. Accessed 21 Aug 2022
5. Lewis B [*sic*], Clarke H (1878) The cortical lamination of the motor area of the brain. Proc R Soc Lond 27:38–49
6. Lewis B (1878–1879) On the comparative structure of the cortex cerebri. Brain 1:79–96
7. Bevan Lewis W (1882) The Human Brain. Histological and Coarse Methods

of Research. A Manual for Students and Asylum Officers. London: J. and A. Churchill.

8. Bevan Lewis W (1889) A Text-book of Mental Diseases: with Special Reference to the Pathological Aspects of Insanity. London: Charles Griffin.

9. Bevan-Lewis W (1909) The Presidential Address on the Biological Factor in Heredity, delivered at the Sixty-eighth Annual Meeting of the Medico-Psychological Association, held at Wakefield on July 2nd and 23rd, 1909. J Ment Sci 55:591–630

10. Bolton JS (1930) William Bevan-Lewis, M.Sc., M.R.C.S., L.R.C.P. J Ment Sci 76:383–388

11. Hoole DDJ (2013) William Bevan Lewis and the scientific asylum. Newsletter R Coll Psychiatr 10:1–2

12. Wallis J (2017) Investigating the Body in the Victorian Asylum. Doctors, Patients, and Practices. London: Palgrave Macmillan, pp. 164–170

Herbert Coddington Major (1850–1921)

Herbert Coddington Major was a pioneer in the field of neuropathology and comparative neurology in the late 19th century. No previous biographical article devoted to him has been found, suggesting that he is now almost totally, yet unjustifiably, forgotten.

He was born in the Channel Islands. The baptism record for Herbert Coddington Mauger [sic] in St Helier, Jersey, gives his date of birth as 30th January 1850 (St Helier baptisms 1842–1909 Martin to Mauger – Jerripedia (theislandwiki.org)), whereas his marriage entry, as Major, at St. Brelade's Church, Jersey, on 20th February 1906 says "(Born abt 1850)" (St Brelade groom marriages – M – Jerripedia (theislandwiki.org)). His obituary notice in the *BMJ* says that he died on 13th September 1921 [1]. This also records his early education in Jersey before undertaking his medical studies in Edinburgh, then the foremost medical school in the United Kingdom, where he graduated in 1871 and gained a gold medal in 1875 for his thesis (of 67 pages) entitled *Histology of the brain in apes,*

By this time Major was working at the West Riding Pauper Lunatic Asylum at Wakefield, Yorkshire, having been appointed Clinical Assistant (1871) and then Assistant Medical Officer (1872) by the asylum superintendent, James Crichton-Browne (1840–1938) [2], who was then developing the institution into a significant school for neuroscientific research [3]. From an early stage Major took an interest in brain pathology, using the dedicated pathological laboratory facilities which Crichton-Browne had developed at the Wakefield Asylum, and facilitated by the fact that even junior Assistant Medical Officer posts were combined with that of Pathologist. In August 1872, at the Psychological Section of the British Medical Association annual meeting, Crichton-Browne showed "some beautifully prepared sections of Brain-Structure in Health and Disease, the work of Dr. Herbert C. Major, of the West Riding Asylum" (*BMJ* 1872;2:221). Major was an early advocate for staining procedures on brain tissue [4], at a time when most asylum post-mortem brain examinations were simply macroscopic.

Major was a significant contributor to the asylum house journal, the *West Riding Lunatic Asylum Medical Reports* (henceforward *WRLAMR*), published annually between 1871 and 1876. He authored six papers in all between 1872 and 1876, more than any other contributor save Crichton-Browne himself [5]. These works ranged from single detailed case studies ("On the minute structure of the cortical substance of the brain, in a case of chronic brain wasting"), through case series ("Observations on the histology of the brain in the insane" and "Observations on the histology of the morbid brain"), to more technical papers ("A new method of determining the depth of the grey matter of the cerebral convolutions"). The latter paper, published in 1872, used an instrument of his own design, the tephrylometer, to measure the thickness of the grey matter. Crichton-Browne also exhibited this "ingenious glass instrument" at the August 1872 BMA meeting.

Lest it be thought he spent all his timing gazing down a microscope, it is also clear that Major did his share of clinical work at the asylum. He undertook most of the work on which Clifford Allbutt's *WRLAMR* paper "The electric treatment of the insane" was based, and Crichton-Browne used his clinical notes on a patient with puerperal mania, pelvic haematocele, and sudden death for a report in the *Lancet* (1874;1:54). Major was also present at some of the annual medical *conversazione* held at the asylum (e.g. 1872, 1873, 1874, and 1875) presiding over stalls showing microscopic preparations from the asylum collection. He also gave lectures on Mental Diseases at the Leeds School of Medicine, a role initiated by Crichton-Browne.

As indicated by the subject matter of his thesis, Major's interests extended beyond the human brain. He had a particular interest in "The histology of the island of Reil," the subject of his final paper in *WRLAMR*, and performed a comparative study of this structure in apes [6]. In these works he may have described, *avant le nom*, the spindle-shaped neurones subsequently described by and later named for Constantin von Economo [7]. John Hunter Arbuckle, a former Clinical Assistant at Wakefield Asylum, later described Major as "the first authority on the minute structure of the cerebral cortex of man and monkeys" [8]. In addition to examining senile atrophy in the human brain, Major also examined ageing dog, horse, and cat brains in search of analogous changes, as reported in his penultimate *WRLAMR* paper "On the morbid histology of the brain in the lower animals". Subsequent comparative studies included an examination of the brain of a Chacma baboon (1875–6) obtained from the Zoological Gardens, London [9], and of a white (beluga) whale obtained from the Westminster Aquarium [10].

After Crichton-Browne's resignation from the Wakefield asylum superintendency in late 1875, Major was appointed in his place in early 1876. It was a hard act to follow. Major co-edited the sixth volume of *WRLAMR* but did not continue the journal, its termination presaging the emergence of *Brain* in 1878 (to which Major did not contribute). Another aspect of Major's "inheritance" was the probability that further asylum accommodation would be needed in the West Riding due to the apparent increase in lunacy. This may have stimulated his interest in statistical tables of the causes of insanity [11], a scheme which spread to asylums nationally later in the following decade [12].

The administrative burdens of asylum superintendency seem to have weighed heavily on Major. Although he still published occasional case reports with detailed neuropathological correlation (e.g. [13]), these were fewer. He resigned the superintendency in 1884. As the *Journal of Mental Science* (1884–1885;30:654) noted, "Dr. Major has ... by his individual efforts in varied histological research advanced science *pari passu* with the fulfilment of the routine duties of administration, although unfortunately at the sacrifice of his health." His successor as superintendent at Wakefield was William Bevan-Lewis (1847–1929), also a noted neuropathologist.

Major was later able to resume clinical work, as a consulting physician at the Infirmary in Bradford, before moving to Bedford, then back to Jersey where he was married to Mary Ann Balleine in 1906. He had recently moved to Oxford at the time of his death [1]. Some 10 years afterwards, the Medical Charitable Society for the West Riding of the County of York received a legacy of £500 under the terms of the will of the late Mrs. M.A. Major "in memory of her husband, Dr. Herbert Coddington Major, formerly of the West Riding Asylum" (*BMJ* 1931;2:270–1).

Acknowledgement

Adapted from: Larner AJ. Herbert Coddington Major (1850–1921). *J Neurol* 2024;271:2144–2146.

References

1. Anon. H C Major M.D., Consulting Physician, Bradford Royal Infirmary. BMJ 1921;2:542.
2. Cambiaghi M. James Crichton-Browne (1840–1938). J Neurol 2019;266:1819–1820.
3. Finn MA. The West Riding Lunatic Asylum and the making of the modern brain sciences in the nineteenth century. Unpublished PhD thesis, University of Leeds. 2012. https://etheses.whiterose.ac.uk/3412/ (accessed 29/11/23).
4. Major HC. The value of the staining process in the histology of the morbid brain. Lancet 1874;1:333–334.
5. Larner AJ. The *West Riding Lunatic Asylum Medical Reports* – the precursor of *Brain*? Brain 2023;146:4437–4445.
6. Major HC. The structure of the island of Reil in apes. Lancet 1877;2:45–46, 84–85.
7. Larner AJ, Triarhou LC. Herbert Major on the insula: an early depiction of von Economo neurones? J Chem Neuroanat 2024;138:102435.
8. Arbuckle JH. A rapid and simple method of staining and mounting fresh brain for microscopic examination. Glasgow Med J 1876;8:207–212.
9. Major HC. Observations on the brain of the Chacma Baboon. J Ment Sci 1875–1876;21:498–512.

10. Major HC. Observations on the structure of the brain of the white whale (*Delphinapterus leucas*). J Anat Physiol 1879;13:127–138.1.
11. Major HC. On statistical tables of the causes of insanity. J Psychol Med Ment Pathol (Lond) 1877;3:260–264.
12. Major HC. Remarks on the results of the collective record of the causation of insanity. J Ment Sci 1884–1885;30:1–7.
13. Major HC. Case of paralytic idiocy with right-sided hemiplegia; epilepsy; atrophy with sclerosis of the left hemisphere of the cerebrum and of the right lobe of the cerebellum. J Ment Sci 1879–1880;25:161–165.

Arthur Thomas Myers (1851–1894): "Quaerens", "Z", and "Dr. Z" revisited

Abstract

John Hughlings Jackson (1835–1911), the foremost English clinical neurologist of the late nineteenth century, made inferences about the workings of the central nervous system in health and disease based on close study of patients' symptoms. Amongst his many publications, he presented two patients with epileptic seizures, both medical men, using pseudonyms: "Quaerens" and "Z". "Dr. Z", as he later came to be called, and considered to be a paradigm case of temporal lobe epilepsy, was identified many years after Jackson's death as Arthur Thomas Myers (1851–1894). Some distinguished historians of neurology have claimed that Quaerens and Z/Myers are in fact the same person. Here the historical record is re-examined, leading to the conclusion that, despite the affirmations of established authorities, Quaerens and Z were not the same individual. This judgment is based on the date of onset of their seizures as reported by the patients themselves, and the dates when they were first seen by Hughlings Jackson as reported by Jackson. The purpose of this paper is not only to serve as a corrective but also to seek reasons to try to explain how this misidentification has become embedded in the secondary literature. In this regard, the misdating by Hughlings Jackson of a publication by Quaerens describing his seizures, a dating apparently accepted as correct by some later authors, may be significant.

Introduction

In the issue of the *British Medical Journal* (henceforward *BMJ*) of 13th January 1894, the following note appeared:

> WE regret to announce the death of Dr. A. T. Myers, Physician to the Belgrave Hospital for Children, and late Medical Registrar of St. George's Hospital, which occurred at his residence, No. 2, Manchester Square, on the morning of January 10th. Dr. Myers, who was well known by his researches into medico-psychological problems, had been in failing health for many months. Dr. Myers was among our oldest and most valued contributors. (*BMJ* 1894;1:94) [capitals in original].

The obituary for "Arthur Thomas Myers, M.A., M.D. Cantab., F.R.C.P." was published in the *BMJ* issue of 27ᵗʰ January 1894. It noted that he died at the early age of 42 and, after listing his intellectual and sporting achievements, commented:

> Nature had, indeed, worthily designed him as one of those good "all round men" who are the glory of our public school education; but destiny thought fit to inflict upon him that terrible and inscrutable nervous malady which occasionally harassed him in early youth, and of late years advanced with relentless tread, baffling the most devoted medical skill, and ultimately involving a fine intellect in ruin and confusion. There can be no doubt but for this Myers would have obtained the highest medical distinction. (*BMJ* 1894;1:223).

The "terrible and inscrutable nervous malady" that afflicted Myers, the name of which could not be written here, was epilepsy. Despite this, Myers has become one of the classic cases in the history of clinical epileptology.

The historical record

Around twenty years before Myers' death, a correspondent under the pseudonym of "Quaerens" (a Latin word meaning seeking, looking for, asking, questioning, inquiring) had written a personal account of a seizure disorder which was published in the May 1870 issue of *The Practitioner: A Journal of Therapeutics*. Following pertinent quotations from the works of Coleridge, Tennyson, and Dickens, Quaerens wrote:

> Last year I had the misfortune to become, for the first time in my life, subject to occasional epilepsy. I well remember that the sensation above described [in the quotation from Dickens's *David Copperfield*, suggestive of déjà vu], with which I had been familiar from boyhood, had, shortly before my first seizure at a time of over-work, become more intense and more frequent than usual. Since my first attack, I have had only few recurrences of the feeling in question. On two occasions, however, it was followed next day by an epileptic seizure, and I have since treated its occurrence as an indication for immediate rest and treatment.
>
> There seems to me a twofold therapeutic interest in this experience. First that, whatever pretty suggestions Coleridge and Tennyson may make to account for it, and however universal its occurrence may be regarded by Dickens, it probably ought to be regarded as showing disturbance of brain-function; and that, perhaps, its recognition and removal might sometimes prevent the development of a more important disorder. Secondly, that inquiry in cases of epilepsy may detect a something of this sort, put aside

as not being of sufficient consequence to speak of; and yet in truth being a minimised form of *petit mal*, warning to precautions against a larger seizure. [1]

Quaerens' publication subsequently came to the attention of Dr John Hughlings Jackson (1835–1911), perhaps the pre-eminent clinician with an interest in epilepsy at this time. In a paper published in *Brain* in July 1880, having mentioned the writings of Coleridge, Tennyson, and Dickens, Jackson wrote in a footnote:

> Quotations are given from these authors by Quaerens, a medical man, who reports his own case – epileptic attacks beginning by "reminiscence" – in *The Practitioner*, May 1870. [2]

As there is more information in this footnote than can be confidently inferred from Quaerens' original publication, namely his occupation, it is possible that Hughlings Jackson knew, or knew of, Quaerens. As pointed out by Greenblatt [3], Jackson's recent biographer, the editor of *The Practitioner* was Francis Anstie, the brother-in-law of Hughlings Jackson's colleague and friend, Thomas Buzzard. In fact, as a later publication was to reveal, Quaerens was by this time Hughlings Jackson's patient.

Quaerens' publication was cited again by Hughlings Jackson in his paper on the "dreamy state" published in *Brain* in July 1888, giving "the whole of the patient's report of his own case" (the two paragraphs cited above) and opining that this was "the first definite case of epilepsy with that phenomenon ('dreamy state') published in this country" [4]. Moreover, further clinical details were now given by Jackson:

> I refer also to the case of a medical man who reported it [slight fits] himself under the pseudonym Quaerens (*Practitioner*, May 1874 [*sic*], p.284). The title is, "A Prognostic and Therapeutical [*sic*] Indication in Epilepsy." When he consulted me, Feb. 1880, he had had eighteen severe fits (loss of consciousness, convulsion, tongue-biting), and had had "many hundreds" of slight attacks. The *slight* attacks which he still had when I first saw him, were so slight that strangers noticed nothing wrong with him; he is never quite unconscious in them; the severest of these slight fits only "bemaze" him for a minute or two; he can go on talking. [4] [italics in original]

It is to be noted that Hughlings Jackson erred here with respect to Quaerens' original publication, in both the title ("therapeutical" rather than "therapeutic") and, more importantly, the year of publication (1874, rather than 1870). Some later authors have interpreted this dating as a correction of Jackson's 1880 *Brain* paper footnote, rather than, in actuality, the introduction of error.

Hughlings Jackson's 1888 *Brain* paper reported on "about fifty cases" of this "particular variety of epilepsy", the "dreamy state", with a number of other case histories besides that of Quaerens included in the text. One of these was first alluded to immediately before the above quoted details about Quaerens, thus:

> One of my patients (*vide infra*, Case 5), a medical man, had seizures of this variety of epilepsy in so slight a degree at first, that he took no more notice of them than to make them a subject of joking (to use the words from the report he made of his own case, he "regarded the matter playfully, as of no practical importance"). He now has severe as well as slight fits. [4]

The final six pages of Jackson's 1888 paper were devoted to the account written by "Case 5" which he dates from July 1888. This account begins:

> I first noticed symptoms which I subsequently learnt to describe as *petit-mal* when living at one of our universities, 1871. [4]

Having followed up this patient, Jackson gave more details on his case in a further *Brain* publication some ten years later, 1898, now referring to him, for the first time, using the pseudonym "Z":

> I first saw the patient, a medical man, whom I call Z, in December 1877. He was then 26 years of age. He began to have slight epileptic attacks in 1871; they were so slight at first that he, to use his own words, "regarded the matter playfully and as of no practical importance." In 1874, he had a *haut-mal*, and then for the first time knew the evil meaning of the slight seizures he had disregarded. He afterwards wrote out for me an account of his case, which, with his consent, I published (*Brain*, Pt. xlii, July 1888, pp. 201 *et seq.*). [5]

This patient had died in January 1894. At post mortem, the pathologist, Walter Stacy Colman (1864–1934), found a very small area of softening in the left uncinate gyrus with a small cavity below the surface just in front of the recurved tip of the uncus [5,6]. This pathological finding prompted Hughlings Jackson's use of the terminology "uncinate fits" for this variety of epilepsy.

An overview of the historical record summarising the complicated chronology of the primary literature relating to Arthur Myers, Quaerens, Z, and Dr.Z, is presented in Table 1.

Who's who? One patient or two?

So what is the relationship between Arthur Thomas Myers, Quaerens, and Z? A number of accounts have appeared in the secondary literature (Table 2), which do not all agree with one another, nor with the historical record. An overview of these accounts may assist in the following attempt to disentangle the various claims.

Because Hughlings Jackson had reported that Z died in January 1894 [5], Taylor & Marsh examined contemporary obituaries in the medical press and were thus able to identify for the first time, in 1980, that Z, who they called "Dr. Z", was Arthur Thomas Myers (1851–1894) [7]. They cited the *BMJ* notice of death, given above, and the subsequent *BMJ* obituary *in toto*. According to Greenblatt [3], the name "Dr. Z" was not used in print by Jackson. Taylor & Marsh made no mention of Quaerens in their paper identifying "Dr. Z".

Kenneth Dewhurst, writing on Hughlings Jackson and psychiatry in 1982, credited E.M. Thornton as "the first to point out that 'Quaerens' and 'Dr. Z' were the same person" [8]. Thornton had claimed in 1976 that "Early in 1874 [*sic*] Hughlings Jackson was attracted by an item in the *Practitioner* ... by an anonymous physician who signed himself "Quaerans" [*sic*]". Accordingly, "Intrigued by this item, Jackson contacted the anonymous physician and asked him to write a full account of his case. He followed him until his death several years later from an overdose of chloral" [9]. Hence Thornton misdated Quaerens' publication (and also, in the bibliography, the volume: 12 instead of 4). Furthermore, Thornton conflated Quaerens with Z: although noting Quaerens' report of symptoms from "boyhood" [1], the onset of symptoms was also stated to be "at the university in 1871", as reported in the account by Z published by Jackson in 1888 [4]. Thornton did not mention Z by name, although both of Hughlings Jackson's *Brain* papers relating to him appeared in the bibliography [9]. Taylor & Marsh made no reference Thornton's book which predated their publication [7].

Although Thornton had made no explicit identification of Quaerens and Z, the implicit identification based on the elision of two separate accounts was subsequently endorsed by Dewhurst on the grounds that in Z's account "are the exact words used earlier by 'Quaerens'" [8]. The specific example Dewhurst cited was Z's report concerning the onset of his symptoms of epilepsy "as of no practical importance". This wording occurs twice in Jackson's 1888 *Brain* paper [4] but on both occasions it relates to "Case 5" (i.e. Z); it is not found in Quaerens' account (original or quoted by Jackson), although Quaerens wrote of symptoms which might be deemed as "not being of sufficient consequence to speak of" [1]. In his bibliography Dewhurst erred in the date (1874), volume (8) and title ("A prognosis...") of Quaerens' publication.

Macdonald and Eileen Critchley, in their 1998 biography of Hughlings Jackson [10], implicitly dated Quaerens' paper to 1874 (i.e. appearing two years before another paper which they discuss which was published in 1876) but did not give a citation for Quaerens' paper. They wrote that Quaerens "was later spoken of under the sobriquet of 'Dr. Z', but eventually it was realised that he was actually Dr. Alfred [sic] Thomas Meyers [sic], a physician at the Belgrave Hospital in London". Their index entry for Quaerens advises "See also 'Dr. Z'" but this entry leads back to Quaerens, likewise the index entry for "Meyers, A.T.". They mentioned that "the case was written up" by Dewhurst and by Taylor & Marsh [10].

Hogan & Kaiboriboon, writing in 2003, stated that "In 1870, Dr. Z, writing under the pseudonym Quaerens (the seeker), published a brief article quoting Coleridge, Tennyson, and Dickens to describe his symptoms. Dr. Z wrote detailed descriptions of his own seizures, reported by Hughlings-Jackson [sic] in 1888. Eventually it was determined that Dr. Z was actually Dr. Alfred [sic] Thomas Meyers [sic], a physician at the Belgrave Hospital in London, with whom Hughlings-Jackson was acquainted" [11]. In their reference section, they give the correct date of Quaerens' publication (1870) but the wrong journal volume (3, rather than 4).

Alastair Compston gave the chronology of patient Z/Dr. Z and then wrote: "Another medical man (to be known as 'Quaerens') who consulted Jackson in February 1880 likened his own symptoms to the state of reminiscence" [12].

Lardreau, discussing the dreamy state, gives a footnote citing Hogan & Kaiboriboon to the effect that the patient is "Alfred Thomas Meyer [sic]" [13].

Samuel H. Greenblatt stated that "There are three names for the same person: (1) Quaerens, (2) Jackson's Z, and (3) A.T. Myers" [3]. Elsewhere he referenced Thornton's book but did not ascribe the identity of Quaerens and Z to this work. In his bibliography Greenblatt erred in the date (1874) and volume (3) of Quaerens' publication. His index entries for "Myers, A.T." and "Z" direct the reader to "Quaerens".

Simon Shorvon stated that "in 1880, Jackson described the clinical semiology in a patient (a medical doctor with the pseudonym 'Querens' [sic]), who committed suicide ten years later and came to post-mortem". In a footnote he credited Taylor and Marsh for the "brilliant piece of detective work" which identified "Hughlings Jackson's Dr Z" [14]. The evident implication here is that Shorvon has identified 'Querens' and "Dr Z" to be the same person.

Discussion

If the material presented here seems a tangle, if not a Gordian knot, to the reader, then it initially appeared so to the writer, hence this exercise as "medical detective" to untangle matters. The work thus produced does not fit easily into the genre of either clinical medicine or literary history. Nevertheless, there are lessons to be learned from a consideration of the material.

Hughlings Jackson's patient "Dr. Z" has been described as the "paradigm of temporal lobe epilepsy" [7] and as having "played a central role in Hughlings-Jackson's [sic] descriptions and understanding of the 'dreamy state'" [11]. Understanding Z's identity and knowing whether published patient accounts of epilepsy emanate from him or from other patients is therefore more than merely an academic issue.

There is no doubt of the identity of Z with Arthur Thomas Myers, as established by Taylor & Marsh in 1980 [7]. However, the question remains as to whether or not Quaerens is the same person as Z. If it were the case that Quaerens is Z, this begs the question as to why Jackson felt the need to invent a second pseudonym, "Z", in 1898 for someone already known as Quaerens based on the self-report of 1870 and in Jackson's papers of 1880 and 1888. Nevertheless, some authorities on Jackson and his work have explicitly or implicitly made this identification: chronologically, Dewhurst [8]; the Critchleys [10]; Hogan & Kaiboriboon [11]; Greenblatt [3]; and Shorvon [13]; whereas others are clear that Quaerens and Z are separate individuals: Compston [12]. Unpicking this knot is complicated, but not impossible: the key facts from the historical record are the dates of seizure onset as reported by the patients themselves, and the dates of first consultation as reported by Jackson (Table 1).

From the historical record, in May 1870 Quaerens reported his episodes had begun in "boyhood" and his epileptic seizures had onset "last year", hence 1869 [1]. This was two years before the onset of Z's first symptoms in 1871, and five years before Z's first "*haut-mal*" in 1874, according to Z's own report [4]. As this self-report was written in 1888, some years after the events he was recalling, Z's precise datings might possibly have been mistaken, but even were this so it is inconceivable that he could have written the paper published in 1870 "under the pseudonym Quaerens" [11] when, as he was born in 1851, he would have been aged only 18 or 19, and still an undergraduate.

In addition to the discrepancies in time of symptom onset in the respective self-reports of Quaerens and Z, Hughlings Jackson also reported different times for his first consultation with the two medical men: Quaerens in February 1880 [4], and Z in December 1877 [5]. It seems highly unlikely that Jackson, meticulous in his recording of clinical details, if not in his reference citation skills, was in error here. Dewhurst noted this discrepancy in the reported dates of first consultation but, following his belief in the identity of Quaerens and Z, stated that "Differences in the dates may be explained by the fact that Jackson referred to their first meeting in 1877, but he did not begin to treat him until three years later" [8]. In his paraphrase of Dewhurst, Greenblatt suggested that he

[Dewhurst] had interpreted Jackson's remark about Quaerens "when he consulted me, Feb. 1880" to mean "[first] consulted me" and so he [Dewhurst] concluded that Quaerens became Jackson's patient in 1880, but Jackson's latter statement simply meant "visited me [again]" [3]. If this sounds tortuous, it is – the simpler explanation is surely that Jackson saw two different patients at two different times. Moreover, in his 1888 *Brain* paper, having introduced "One of my patients (*vide infra*, Case 5), a medical man", Jackson was explicit in stating "I refer *also* to the case of a medical man ... under the pseudonym Quaerens" [4] [my italics]. Compston correctly noted that Quaerens was "another medical man" [12].

Hence, Quaerens and Z are different individuals, albeit both medical men, and both afflicted with similar seizure types. How, then, have established authorities in the history of epilepsy and the historiography of Hughlings Jackson previously made an incorrect identification? I suggest that Thornton implicitly misidentified the two by conflating their separate accounts, and that Dewhurst misinterpreted this as an explicit identification when claiming that Thornton was "the first to point out that 'Quaerens' and 'Dr. Z' were the same person" [8]. The Critchleys seem to have followed Dewhurst, for example in the misdating of Quaerens' paper as 1874 rather than 1870. The elision of Quaerens, Z, and Myers made by Greenblatt also appears to stem from the misdating of Quaerens' publication. This paper appeared in May 1870 [1], as per the footnote in Hughlings Jackson's July 1880 *Brain* paper [2], not in 1874 as stated in Hughlings Jackson's July 1888 *Brain* paper [4]. But Greenblatt states that in his 1880 paper "Jackson gives the date of Quaerens' piece *incorrectly as 1870*" [my italics]; accordingly, Greenblatt's chronology of Quaerens begins in May 1874, rather than in May 1870 [3]. I infer that Greenblatt may have followed the Critchleys in this misdating, since he noted their misspelling of "Meyers" for Myers (but not of "Alfred" for Arthur). The identical errors in the naming of Z (as "Alfred" and "Meyers") may suggest that Hogan & Kaiboriboon [11] have followed the Critchleys, although how they arrived at the view that Dr. Z initially "wrote under the pseudonym Quaerens" is unclear, as they cite no sources; it might possibly stem from Dewhurst's interpretation, although they do not cite him. Shorvon provides no documentary evidence that Quaerens committed suicide; moreover, Z died, intentionally or accidentally, in 1894, not in 1890 as implied in his account [13].

A pertinent question in light of these findings is to ask how this misidentification has persisted, with the honourable exception of Compston's paper [12], in the secondary literature for over 40 years? Perhaps the various authors did not view the original Quaerens paper (it may now be viewed online) but relied on the earlier, incorrect, citations, hence perpetuating error. However, the full text of Quaerens' publication is repeated by Jackson in his 1888 *Brain* paper, although he then misdated the original publication [4]. Searching for the original Quaerens' paper using the citation details in the secondary sources first alerted me to the concatenation of errors outlined above.

The corollary of this deidentification of Quaerens and Z is that the identity of Quaerens remains unknown. In the absence of Hughlings Jackson's papers, destroyed at his death as per his instruction, Quaerens' identity may never be established. We are still seeking.

Addendum: now and then

As specified in the *BMJ* notice of his death, Myers' address was "No. 2, Manchester Square", hence adjacent to Hughlings Jackson, who lived at No.3. Jackson was therefore able to arrange the post-mortem examination, although this was not published until 1898. Myers shared the tenancy of the house with Dr. Frederick Dawtrey Drewitt (1848–1942), who had also once worked at the Belgrave Hospital. (He later wrote a biography of Edward Jenner [15].)

Z's account of his seizures, published by Hughlings Jackson, contains a remarkable example of amnesia:

> I was attending a young patient whom his mother had brought me with some history of lung symptoms. I wished to examine the chest, and asked him to undress on a couch. I thought he looked ill, but have no recollection of any intention to recommend him to take to his bed at once, or of any diagnosis. Whilst he was undressing I felt the onset of a petit mal. I remember taking out my stethoscope and turning away a little to avoid conversation. The next thing I recollect is that I was sitting at a writing table in the same room, speaking to another person, and as my consciousness became more complete, recollected my patient, but saw he was not in the room. I was interested to ascertain what had happened, and had an opportunity an hour later of seeing him in bed with a note of a diagnosis I had made of "pneumonia of the left base." I gathered indirectly from conversation that I had made a physical examination, written these words, and advised him to take to bed at once. I re-examined him with some curiosity, and found that my conscious diagnosis was the same as my unconscious, – or perhaps I should say, unremembered diagnosis had been. I was a good deal surprised, but not so unpleasantly as I should have thought probable [4].

Accordingly, Z has been noted as one of the earliest accounts of amnesia in temporal lobe epilepsy [16], and perhaps the first reported or index case of transient epileptic amnesia (TEA), a rare syndrome characterised by brief, repeated episodes of amnesia, often occurring on waking, and sometimes accompanied by other automatisms [17,18]. Although magnetic resonance brain imaging in most of these cases is reported to be normal [18], in occasional cases swelling of the medial temporal lobe may be seen which sometimes resolves with control of the seizures [19–21]. It has been suggested [21], with caveats, that these neuroradiological findings might be the neuroimaging correlate of the neuropathological findings first described in "Z" in 1898 by Hughlings Jackson and Colman [5], but sadly these authors also fell into the trap of equating Quaerens and Z [21].

As for Myers' role as "among our oldest and most valued contributors", he did publish a paper in the *BMJ* in 1886, on smallpox [22], the abstract of a paper read before the Clinical Society of London (and also published in its *Transactions*; see Taylor & Marsh, 1980:765, for a brief Myers' bibliography). Myers' affiliation is listed in the *BMJ* paper as "Late Medical Registrar to St. George's Hospital". He also had a publication in the *Journal of Mental Science* on a celebrated case of multiple personality, Louis V [23], a case which his brother, Frederic, one of the founder members of the British Society for Psychical Research, also published on (Frederic Myers elsewhere acknowledged his indebtness to the work of Hughlings Jackson on affections of speech and the evolution and dissolution of the nervous system [24]). AT Myers also had a publication in *Nature* on a medical index-catalogue [25]. He contributed the article on "Hypnotism, History of" to Hack Tuke's 1892 *Dictionary of Psychological Medicine* [26]. He was appointed FRCP in 1893 but as a consequence of his epilepsy had to give up clinical practice in October of that year; in the same year he began living in the same house as Dawtrey Drewitt.

However, it is clear that Arthur Thomas Myers is remembered by posterity as a patient rather than as a clinician, by his anonym "Z" rather than by his real name. He was a seeker, but he was not "Quaerens".

Acknowledgement

Unpublished manuscript, early 2024.

References

1. Quaerens. A prognostic and therapeutic indication in epilepsy. *The Practitioner* 1870; 4: 284–5. https://archive.org/details/practitioner04londuoft/page/n5/mode/2up
2. Jackson JH. On right or left-sided spasm at the onset of epileptic paroxysms and on crude sensation-warnings and elaborate mental states. *Brain* 1880–1881; 3(2): 192–206. [Reprinted in: Taylor J, Holmes G, Walshe FMR (eds.). *John Hughlings Jackson. Selected Writings. Volume 1. On epilepsy and epileptiform convulsions.* Nijmegen: Arts and Boeve, 1931 [1996]: 308–17].
3. Greenblatt SH. *John Hughlings Jackson. Clinical neurology, evolution, and Victorian brain science.* Oxford: Oxford University Press, 2022.
4. Jackson JH. On a particular variety of epilepsy (intellectual aura). One case with symptoms of organic brain disease. *Brain* 1888; 11: 179–207 [Reprinted

in: Taylor J, Holmes G, Walshe FMR (eds.). *John Hughlings Jackson. Selected Writings. Volume 1. On epilepsy and epileptiform convulsions.* Nijmegen: Arts and Boeve, 1931 [1996]: 385–405].

5. Jackson JH, Colman WS. Case of epilepsy with tasting movements and "dreamy state" – very small patch of softening in the left uncinate gyrus. *Brain* 1898; 21: 580–90. [Reprinted in: Taylor J, Holmes G, Walshe FMR (eds.). *John Hughlings Jackson. Selected Writings. Volume 1. On epilepsy and epileptiform convulsions.* Nijmegen: Arts and Boeve, 1931 [1996]: 458–63].

6. Anon. Epilepsy with lesion of uncinate gyrus. *JAMA* 1899; 32: 1067–8.

7. Taylor DC, Marsh SM. Hughlings Jackson's Dr Z: the paradigm of temporal lobe epilepsy revealed. *J Neurol Neurosurg Psychiatry* 1980; 43: 758–67.

8. Dewhurst K. *Hughlings Jackson on psychiatry.* Oxford: Sandford Publications, 1982: pp. 91–102.

9. Thornton EM. *Hypnotism, hysteria and epilepsy: an historical synthesis.* London: William Heinemann Medical Books, 1976.

10. Critchley M, Critchley EA. *John Hughlings Jackson. Father of English neurology.* Oxford: Oxford University Press, 1998.

11. Hogan RE, Kaiboriboon K. The "dreamy state": John Hughlings-Jackson's [*sic*] ideas of epilepsy and consciousness. *Am J Psychiatry* 2003; 160: 1740–7.

12. Compston A. From the archives. *Brain* 2007; 130: 1712–4.

13. Lardreau E. An approach to nineteenth-century medical lexicon: the term "dreamy state". *J Hist Neurosci* 2011; 20: 34–41.

14. Shorvon S. *The idea of epilepsy. A medical and social history of epilepsy in the modern era (1860-2020).* Cambridge: Cambridge University Press, 2023.

15. Drewitt FD. *The life of Edward Jenner. Naturalist, and discoverer of vaccination.* Cambridge: Cambridge University Press, 1933 [2013].

16. Khalsa SS, Moore SA, Van Hoesen GW. Hughlings Jackson and the role of the entorhinal cortex in temporal lobe epilepsy: from Patient A to Doctor Z. *Epilepsy Behav* 2006; 9: 524–31.

17. Zeman AZJ, Boniface SJ, Hodges JR. Transient epileptic amnesia: a description of the clinical and neuropsychological features in 10 cases and a review of the literature. *J Neurol Neurosurg Psychiatry* 1998; 64: 435–43.

18. Baker J, Savage S, Milton F et al. The syndrome of transient epileptic amnesia: a combined series of 115 cases and literature review. *Brain Commun* 2021; 3: fcab038.

19. Butler CR, Zeman A. A case of transient epileptic amnesia with radiological localization. *Nature Clin Pract Neurol* 2008; 4: 516–21.

20. Larner AJ. Transient epileptic amnesia and amygdala enlargement revisited. *Psychogeriatrics* 2021; 21: 943–4.

21. McGinty RN, Larner AJ. Transient epileptic amnesia and medial temporal lobe swelling: further cases and historical perspective. *J Neurol* 2024; 271: 589–92.

22. Whipham TT, Myers AT. On some chronic nervous sequelae of small-pox, especially as affecting he speech. *BMJ* 1886; 1: 584–6.

23. Myers AT. Psychological retrospect. The life-history of a case of double or multiple personality. *J Ment Sci* 1885–1886; 31 (January 1886): 596–605.
24. Harrington A. *Medicine, mind, and the double brain. A study in Nineteenth-Century thought.* Princeton: Princeton University Press, 1987: 139.
25. Myers AT. A medical index-catalogue. IndexCatalogue of the Library of the Surgeon General's Office. US Army Vol VII Insignares-Leghorn. *Nature* 1886–1887; 35: 196.
26. Myers AT. Hypnotism, History of. In: Tuke DH (ed.). *A dictionary of psychological medicine giving the definition, etymology and synonyms of the terms used in medical psychology with the symptoms, treatment, and pathology of insanity and the law of lunacy in Great Britain and Ireland.* London: J & A Churchill, 1892; I: 603–6.

Table 1: Quaerens and Z: Chronology of events in the primary literature

Month/year	Event	Reference or citation
May 1870	"Quaerens": self-description of epilepsy appears in *The Practitioner*	1
1871	"Z": first experiences *petit mal* whilst an undergraduate by his own account	4, p.201
1874	"Z": first experiences haut mal by his own account	4, p.202
December 1877	"Z": has first consultation with Jackson	5, p.580
February 1880	"Quaerens": has first consultation with Jackson	4, p.184
July 1880	Jackson: in his paper in *Brain*, Jackson first cites Quaerens' *Practitioner* paper, giving the correct date, May 1870	2, p.199n
July 1888	Jackson: in his *Brain* paper, Jackson mentions both Quaerens and "Z" (= "Case 5"); this is the first published report of "Z". JHJ now misdates Quaerens' paper as 1874 (cf. Jackson's July 1880 paper)	5, pp.181, 184–6; 184, 201–207
[10] January 1894	"Z": dies from "overdose of chloral".	5, p.580
27 January 1894	Obituary of Arthur Thomas Myers appears in *BMJ*.	BMJ 1894;1:223
October 1898	Jackson: first use of the pseudonym "Z" in report of post mortem findings (by Colman) published in *Brain*	5, p.580

Table 2: Quaerens and Z: Chronology of events in the secondary literature

Month/year	Event	Reference or citation
1976	Thornton: conflates accounts of "Quaerans" [sic], misdated as 1874, and Z (without using that name), hence implicitly identifying the two	9, p. 29
1980	Taylor & Marsh: identify "Dr. Z" as Arthur Thomas Myers	7
1982	Dewhurst: claims Thornton identified Quaerens and Z as the same person and endorses this, based erroneously on "exact words" used by Z and Quaerens; misdates Quaerens' paper as 1874	8, p.92
1998	Critchleys: Quaerens spoken of as 'Dr. Z', and that it was eventually realised he was "Dr. Alfred Thomas Meyers"; imply Quaerens' paper was 1874	10, pp.68–69
2003	Hogan & Kaiboriboon: claim Dr. Z wrote under seudonym Quaerens in 1870. Identify Z as "Dr. Alfred Thomas Meyers"	11, p.174 1
2007	Compston: correctly differentiates Quaerens and Z	12, p.1713
2022	Greenblatt: equates Quaerens, Jackson's Z, and A.T. Myers; misdates Quaerens' paper as 1874	3, p.446 n222, 518
2023	Shorvon: identifies 'Querens' [sic] with Dr. Z. Implies Quaerens/Dr. Z died in 1890.	14, p.67

Arnold Pick (1851–1924): a centenary appreciation

Introduction

2024 marks the centenary of the death of Arnold Pick (1851–1924). Many clinicians are aware of the name and of "Pick's disease" although they may be unclear exactly who he was or what this terminology designates. This article seeks to give some brief biographical details, recap Pick's key findings on "Pick's disease", and relate the latter to current thinking about the classification of frontotemporal dementia, an undertaking which prompts the consideration as to whether the eponym should stand or be laid to rest as now obsolete and superseded.

Biography[1,2]

Arnold Pick was born in Moravia, a province of the Hapsburg Empire, in 1851. He graduated from the Vienna Medical School in 1875; part of his training was with Theodor Meynert and he overlapped with Carl Wernicke. From the late 1870s he worked mostly in Prague, taking the chair of neuropsychiatry at the German University there in 1886 where he remained chairman until his retirement in 1921.

Pick's many publications covered a wide range of interests, including work on aphasia, wherein he introduced the concept of agrammatism. The influence of John Hughlings Jackson's (1835–1911) work on aphasia may be evidenced by Pick's dedication of his monograph of 1913 on agrammatism, *Die agrammatischen Sprachstörungen; Studien zur psychologischen Grundlegung der Aphasielehre*, to Hughlings Jackson, as "the deepest thinker in neuropathology of the past century".[3] Indeed, Henry Head (1861–1940) was of the view that until Pick's dedication no one had attempted to understand Hughlings Jackson's contribution to the subject of aphasia.[4] Kertesz reported that "Pick had Jackson's portrait on his desk" and that "Jackson wrote about Pick and popularized his work in England" (ref. 2, p.19). However, other than his mention of Pick in a footnote of his 1894 paper "The Factors of Insanities" ("I know of but a single study of re-evolution, a very valuable one by Professor Pick, of Prague"[5]), I am not currently aware of any other Jackson reference to Pick (he does not appear in Greenblatt's book on Jackson[6]). Alexander Luria[7] credited Pick with recognising the manifestations of afferent apraxia shortly after the original description by Liepmann (1905), citing his *Studien über motorische Aphasie* published in Vienna in 1905.

Pick's publications were by no means limited to behavioural neurology or dementia, nor to the Germanophone literature. He appeared several times in the pages of *Brain*,[8-10] including a description of reduplicative paramnesia.[9] Indeed, his final paper, "On the pathology of echographia", appeared in *Brain* in 1924 with the by-line "By the late A. Pick. Professor in the German University, Prague",[10] indicating that he continued to write until shortly before his death.

Key papers on focal atrophy

Pick published several papers in the late 19th and early 20th centuries describing clinical deficits in association with focal brain atrophy, papers which have been critically discussed.[11-13] These deficits were either linguistic or behavioural in nature.

The first of these papers, dating to 1892, described a man of 71 ("August H.") with progressive aphasia who at post-mortem was found to have marked atrophy of the cortical gyri of the left temporal lobe.[14] Pick reported further cases of language disturbance in association with either frontotemporal atrophy (1901),[15] or left temporal lobe atrophy (1904).[16] By contrast, a patient with behavioural disturbance (apathy, disinhibition, personal neglect) in association with bilateral frontal atrophy was reported in 1906.[17]

Pick was primarily interested in clinico-anatomical correlation and did not report microscopic pathological findings in any of these cases. Indeed, it was Alois Alzheimer (1864–1915), not Pick, who in 1911 described the histological findings in such cases (the name "Pick's disease" was not introduced until the 1920s). Alzheimer specifically described the argyrophilic intracytoplasmic inclusions ("Pick bodies") and the diffusely staining ballooned neurones ("Pick cells") which may be associated with some cases of focal lobar atrophy.[18] (Incidentally, I cannot immediately think of any other instance in which microscopic neuropathological abnormalities have acquired the eponym of someone who had no role in their initial description, but I stand open to correction on this point.) This nomenclature is perhaps all the more surprising in light of the reported rivalry between the laboratories of Alzheimer (in Emil Kraepelin's department) and Pick, which may have been one reason for Kraepelin's promotion of "Alzheimer's disease" as of the 1910 edition (8th) of his textbook of psychiatry.[19]

Judgment of posterity?

Perhaps only those dedicated to the study of the dementias in general and of the frontotemporal lobar degenerations in particular will keep abreast of the different classifications which have been proposed for these disorders.

Previously lumped together as "Pick's disease", this latter terminology has steadily become more marginalised. If used at all now, "Pick's disease" denotes one subtype of frontotemporal lobar degeneration characterised by the neuropathological finding of Pick bodies and Pick cells. A necessary corollary of this formulation is that "Pick's disease" is not, and cannot be, an exclusively clinical diagnosis.

The heterogeneity of the frontotemporal lobar degenerations defined at clinical, pathological, and genetic levels[20] has been responsible for this marginalisation of Pick. An attempt to encompass all these conditions under the rubric of "Pick complex"[21] (i.e. as interrelated variants on the same spectrum, including frontal lobe dementia with or without motor neurone disease, corticobasal degeneration, and primary progressive aphasia) cannot be said to have prospered in the 25 years since its proposal. Current molecular classification of frontotemporal dementias categorizes Pick's disease as 3R FTLD-tau, sometimes with coexistent TDP-43 pathology.[22]

Accordingly, the term "Pick's disease" may now be regarded as effectively redundant, in fact obsolete, the moreso if one takes into account the fact that Pick did not describe the characteristic neuropathological findings of "his" disease. If so, it will nevertheless remain the case, as pointed out by John Hodges, that the relegation of Pick to a minor place in the terminology of frontotemporal dementia is sad in light of his "monumental contributions".[12] In my clinical experience the terminology persisted only in non-specialist medical parlance (e.g. primary care referrals to the memory or cognitive clinic) and in some old age psychiatry clinics (wherein patients labelled as "Pick's disease" may nonetheless have received treatment with cholinesterase inhibitors!).

Acknowledgement

Adapted from: Larner AJ. Arnold Pick (1851–1924): a centenary appreciation. *Adv Clin Neurosci Rehabil* 2024;22(4):14–15.

References

1.   Todman D. *Arnold Pick (1851–1924)*. J Neurol 2009;256:504–505.
2.   Kertesz A. *Arnold Pick: a historical introduction*. In: Kertesz A, Munoz DG (eds.). *Pick's disease and Pick complex*. New York: Wiley-Liss, 1998:13–21.
3.   Critchley M, Critchley EA. *John Hughlings Jackson. Father of English neurology*. Oxford: Oxford University Press, 1998:124.
4.   Head H. Aphasia and kindred disorders of speech. Cambridge: Cambridge University Press, 1926; I: 30. [Cited in Harrington A. *Medicine, mind, and the double brain. A study in Nineteenth-Century thought*. Princeton: Princeton University Press, 1987: 266.]

5. Taylor J, Holmes G, Walshe FMR (eds.). *John Hughlings Jackson. Selected Writings. Volume 2. Evolution and dissolution of the nervous system. Speech. Various papers, addresses and lectures.* Nijmegen: Arts and Boeve, 1931 [1996]: 412n1.

6. Greenblatt SH. *John Hughlings Jackson. Clinical neurology, evolution, and Victorian brain science.* Oxford: Oxford University Press, 2022.

7. Luria AR. *The working brain. An introduction to neuropsychology.* Harmondsworth: Penguin, 1973:173.

8. Pick A. *On the study of true tumours of the optic nerve.* Brain 1901;24(3): 502–508.

9. Pick A. *Clinical studies.* Brain 1903;26(2):242–267.

10. Pick A. *On the pathology of echographia.* Brain 1924;47(4):417–429.

11. Spatt J. *Arnold Pick's concept of dementia.* Cortex 2003;39:525–531.

12. Hodges J. *Pick's disease: its relationship to progressive aphasia, semantic dementia and frontotemporal dementia.* In: Ames D, Burns A, O'Brien J (eds.). *Dementia* (4th edition). London: Hodder Arnold, 2010:647–658.

13. Roelofs A. *Cerebral atrophy as a cause of aphasia: from Pick to the modern era.* Cortex 2023;165:101–118.

14. Pick A. *Über die Beziehungen der senilen Hirnatrophie zur Aphasie.* Prager Medizinische Wochenschrift 1892;17:165–167. [Translation: Girling DM, Berrios GE. *On the relationship between senile cerebral atrophy and aphasia.* Hist Psychiatry 1994;5:542–547.]

15. Pick A. *Senile Hirnatrophie als Grundlage für Hernderscheinungen.* Wiener Klinische Wochenschrift 1901;14:403–404. [Translation: Girling DM, Marková IS. *Senile atrophy as the basis for focal symptoms.* Hist Psychiatry 1995;6:533–537.]

16. Pick A. *Zur symptomatologie der linksseitigen Schläffenlappenatrophie.* Monatsschrift für Psychiatrie und Neurologie 1904;16(4):378–388. [Translation: Girling DM, Berrios GE. *On the symptomatology of left-sided temporal lobe atrophy.* Hist Psychiatry 1997;8:149–159.]

17. Pick A. *Über einen weiteren symptomenkomplex im Rahmen der Dementia senilis, bedingt durch umschriebene stärkere Hirnatrophie (gemischte Apraxie).* Monatsschrift für Psychiatrie und Neurologie 1906;19(2):97–108.

18. Alzheimer A. *Über eigenartige Krankheitsfälle des späteren Alters.* Zeitschrift für gesamte Neurologie und Psychiatrie 1911;4:356–385. [Translation: Förstl H, Levy R. *On certain peculiar diseases of old age.* Hist Psychiatry 1991;2:71–101.]

19. Schwartz MF, Stark JA. *The distinction between Alzheimer's disease and senile dementia: historical considerations.* J Hist Neurosci 1992;1:169–187.

20. Dickerson BC (ed.) *Hodges' Frontotemporal dementia* (2nd edition). Cambridge: Cambridge University Press, 2016.

21. Kertesz A, Munoz DG (eds.). *Pick's disease and Pick complex.* New York: Wiley-Liss, 1998.

22. Mackenzie IRA, Neumann M. *Molecular neuropathology of frontotemporal dementia: insights into disease mechanisms from postmortem studies.* J Neurochem 2016;138(Suppl1):54–70.

William Aldren Turner (1864–1945): epileptologist and "shell-shock" doctor

William Aldren Turner is remembered as both an epileptologist and a "shell-shock" doctor [1–4].

He was born in Edinburgh, the son of William Turner (1832–1916) who at the time was senior demonstrator in Anatomy at the University, later Professor (1867). His paternal grandmother was Margaret Aldren. He studied medicine in Edinburgh, qualifying in 1887, and was house officer there before undertaking postgraduate studies in Berlin and at St Bartholomew's Hospital, London (where his father had studied medicine). Loughran suggests Turner may have been influenced by Thomas Claye Shaw, lecturer in psychological medicine at Barts, along with other "shell-shock" doctors such as William H.R. Rivers and Charles S. Myers ([5], p.48).

Turner gained the MRCP in 1889. In 1892 he was appointed assistant to David Ferrier (1843–1928), also an Edinburgh graduate (1868). At this time, Ferrier had been Professor of Forensic Medicine at King's College Hospital since 1872 and full physician there since 1890, as well as physician at the National Hospital for the Paralysed and Epileptic at Queen Square from 1880. Together, Ferrier and Turner undertook animal studies examining the effects of brain lesions, thus continuing Ferrier's experimental work on cortical localisation which he had begun in the early 1870s [6]. Experiments performed under the superintendence of Ferrier formed the basis of Turner's Edinburgh MD thesis of 1892 entitled "Observations on the Anatomy and Physiology of the Central Nervous System" [Papers of William Aldren Turner, 1884–1937 | University of Edinburgh Archive and Manuscript Collections; Observations on the anatomy and physiology of the central nervous system (ed.ac.uk)] which won the gold medal [1] (Ferrier's Edinburgh MD had also won the gold medal, in 1870).

The conjoint studies of Turner and Ferrier were published between 1894 and 1901, specifically related to the cerebellum [7], cerebro-cortical pathways [8] (both of these papers were read at the Royal Society), and the corpora quadrigemina [9] (which had been the subject of Ferrier's MD thesis more than 30 years earlier). In his obituary notice of Ferrier, Turner described him as "the foremost of scientific physicians of his day" (*BMJ* 1928;1:575), but ultimately it was clinical rather than laboratory work that drew Turner. He was elected FRCP in 1896.

There was also evidently clinical collaboration between Turner and Ferrier, since in Turner's chapter on intracranial syphilis in the 1899 textbook *A system of medicine*, edited by Clifford Allbutt, he stated that "I am indebted to Dr. Ferrier for the use of many of the original cases from which the facts stated in this article are taken" [10]. In that year, Turner was appointed assistant physician to King's College Hospital and in 1900 Physician to the National Hospital at Queen Square ([11], p.523).

Turner's major sphere of clinical interest was epilepsy. On this subject he published a series of papers in the *Medico-Chirurgical Transactions* between 1903 and 1905 investigating the prognosis of epilepsy in relation to treatment, "mental condition", and "stigmata of degeneration" [12–14]. These studies, facilitated by the many epilepsy patients he saw both at Queen Square and at the dedicated epilepsy colony at Chalfont St. Peter (opened 1894), where he was visiting physician from 1902 ([15], p.164n4), formed part of the basis for Turner's textbook, *Epilepsy. A study of the idiopathic disease* [16] (the book was misnamed as *"Clinical study of epilepsy"* in his *Lancet* obituary ([2], p.223), although this is a fair description of the contents). This was published in 1907 and dedicated to David Ferrier "in grateful acknowledgment of many acts of kindness". Of particular note, Turner held that by definition convulsions were "frequently accompanied by psychical phenomena" ([16], p.1). He also delivered the Morison Lectures to the Royal College of Physicians of Edinburgh in 1910 on the subject of epilepsy [17]. With Thomas Grainger Stewart (1877–1957) he published *A textbook of nervous diseases* in 1910.

It has been suggested that Turner's work was the first time that "statistical methods" were applied to the study of epilepsy prognosis ([18], p.79), perhaps based on his title [12], but it would perhaps be more correct to say he used numerical rather than statistical methods since beyond percentages and bar-charts there were no available statistical operations such as p values. Later authors have adjudged his epilepsy work as having "consolidated knowledge rather than led to significant advances" [4].

Turner was involved in the setting up of the International League Against Epilepsy (ILAE) in 1909 and presented statistics on epilepsy in the UK at the second ILAE meeting held in Berlin in 1910. He was also on the Comite de la Redaction for the ILAE journal *Epilepsia* ([15], p.11,15,20,21,172).

With the advent of the First World War, Turner was sent to France in December 1914 as "Temporary Lieutenant-Colonel, Royal Army Medical Corps", to investigate reports of soldiers afflicted with nervous and mental shock (this predated C.S. Myers' introduction of the term "shell-shock" in the medical literature in February 1915). Turner noted cases of mental stupor, loss of memory, hearing and visual symptoms, stammering, local palsies and spasms, spinal shock with paraplegia, and neurasthenia [19]. On his return from France, he was instrumental in promoting accommodation of "shell-shock" patients at Queen Square as one of a number of hospitals designated for the reception of soldiers returning from the conflict with unexplained neurological symptoms. Hence, he gained further clinical experience in managing soldiers with "war neurosis" being one of the few Queen Square consultants with first-hand experience from the frontline [20,21]. His Bradshaw Lecture to Royal College of Physicians of London, delivered just four days before the Armistice in November 1918, reiterated many of his initial clinical observations and advocated treatment by segregation in an "atmosphere of cure" provided by special hospitals supplemented with psychotherapy and occupation [22].

This appreciation of the importance of psychological factors in the pathogenesis of neurological symptoms, perhaps first learned from Claye Shaw, manifested in Turner's opinions on epilepsy and reiterated in his management of war neuroses. This viewpoint later informed Turner's Presidential address to the Section of Neurology of the Royal Society of Medicine in 1920 on the "Influence of psychogenic factors in nervous disorders" [23]. (At this time the RSM Section of Neurology was the only dedicated forum for neurology in the UK, as the Association of British Neurologists was not founded until 1932). Turner also contributed to the official *Report of the War Office Committee of Enquiry into "Shell-Shock"* published in 1922 [24]. In that same year, the *King's College Hospital Gazette* reported that he presented to a new student organization, the Neuropathological and Psycho-Pathological Society ([5], pp.230–231).

Turner's wartime experiences continued to influence his civilian practice. At Queen Square, he proposed to the Medical Committee on several occasions the appointment of a "psychotherapeutic officer" but the idea was apparently deferred and then rejected "largely it seems through the influence of [Gordon] Holmes" ([11], p.352). Holmes's response to the war neuroses was quite different from that of Turner [25]. Turner retired from Queen Square in 1925 ([11], p.523, but his date of death is given incorrectly as 1943; also at p.561).

In an appreciation written after his death in July 1945, one of his students ("W.B.") noted of Turner that "His was not a demonstrative nature, but he was always ready to help his students in every way, and to give them opportunities to develop their own interests to the full". He also recalled that "During the last war he showed great foresight and power of appreciation of the psychological factors at work in cases of war neurosis, and with quiet firmness and tenacity helped on the development of new psychological methods in the diagnosis and treatment of functional nervous diseases" [3]. Turner has a memorial tablet in St Luke's Chapel at King's College Hospital.

One of his three sons, John William Aldren Turner (1911–1980) was also a neurologist, who described brachial neuritis (Parsonage-Turner syndrome) in 1948 [26].

Acknowledgements

Adapted and extended from: Larner AJ. William Aldren Turner (1864–1945). J Neurol 2024; 271: 5699–5701.

References

1. Anon. Obituary. W. Aldren Turner, C.B., M.D., F.R.C.P. *BMJ* 1945;2:200.
2. Anon. William Aldren Turner C.B., M.D. EDIN., F.R.C.P. *Lancet* 1945;2:222–223.
3. Anon. The late Dr. W. Aldren Turner. *Lancet* 1945;2:291.
4. Eadie MJ. The epileptology of William Aldren Turner. *J Clin Neurosci* 2006;13:9–13.
5. Loughran T. *Shell-shock and medical culture in First World War Britain.* Cambridge: Cambridge University Press, 2017.
6. Larner AJ. A month in the country: the sesquicentenary of David Ferrier's classical cerebral localisation researches of 1873. *J R Coll Physicians Edinb* 2023;52:128–131.
7. Ferrier D, Turner WA. Record of experiments illustrative of the symptomatology and degenerations following lesions of the cerebellum and its peduncles and related structures in monkeys. *Phil Trans R Soc Lond* 1894;185:719–778.
8. Ferrier D, Turner WA. An experimental research upon cerebro-cortical afferent and efferent tracts. *Phil Trans R Soc Lond* 1898;190:1–44.
9. Ferrier D, Turner WA. Experimental lesion of the corpora quadrigemina in monkeys. *Brain* 1901;24:27–46.
10. Turner WA. Intracranial syphilis. Allbutt C (ed.). *A system of medicine. Volume VII. Diseases of the nervous system (Continued).* London: Macmillan and Co., 1899, pp. 668–685.
11. Shorvon S, Compston A. *Queen Square. A history of the National Hospital and its Institute of Neurology.* Cambridge: Cambridge University Press, 2019.
12. Turner WA. A statistical enquiry into the prognosis and curability of epilepsy based upon the results of treatment. *Med Chir Trans* 1903;86:259–291.
13. Turner WA. The mental condition in epilepsy in relation to prognosis. *Med Chir Trans* 1904;87:349–372.
14. Turner WA. The influence of stigmata of degeneration upon the prognosis of epilepsy. *Med Chir Trans* 1905;88:127–145.
15. Shorvon S, Weiss G, Avanzini G et al. *International League Against Epilepsy 1909-2009. A centenary history.* Chichester: Wiley-Blackwell, 2009:11,15,20,21,172.
16. Turner WA. *Epilepsy. A study of the idiopathic disease.* London: Macmillan and Co., 1907.
17. Turner WA. The Morison Lectures On Epilepsy: delivered before the Royal College of Physicians of Edinburgh. *BMJ* 1910;1:733–737, 803–807, 866–871.
18. Shorvon S. *The idea of epilepsy. A medical and social history of epilepsy in the modern era (1860-2020).* Cambridge: Cambridge University Press, 2023.

19. Turner WA. Remarks on cases of nervous and mental shock observed in the base hospitals in France. *BMJ* 1915;1:833–835.
20. Turner WA. Arrangements for the care of cases of nervous and mental shock coming from overseas. *Lancet* 1916;1:1073–1075.
21. Linden SC, Jones E. "Shell shock" revisited: an examination of the case records of the National Hospital in London. *Med Hist* 2014; 58:519–545.
22. Turner WA. The Bradshaw Lecture on neuroses and psychoses of war. *Lancet* 1918;2:613–617.
23. Turner WA. Influence of psychogenic factors in nervous disorders. *Proc R Soc Med* 1920;13(Neurol Sect):1–16.
24. *Report of the War Office Committee of Enquiry into "Shell-Shock"*. London: HMSO, 1922. Report Of The UK War Office Committee Of Enquiry Into "Shell-Shock" : UK Government : Free Download, Borrow, and Streaming : Internet Archive.
25. Macleod AD. Shell shock, Gordon Holmes and the Great War. *J R Soc Med* 2004;97:86–89.
26. Parsonage MJ, Turner JWA. Neuralgic amyotrophy. The shoulder-girdle syndrome. *Lancet* 1948;1:973–978.

Robert S. Woodworth (1869–1962): his time in Liverpool with Sherrington

More haste less speed

Practice makes perfect

Both these proverbs may be deemed to refer to the trade-off between speed and accuracy which was given empirical support by the studies of the psychologist Robert Woodworth.

Robert Sessions Woodworth demonstrated, in a paper published in 1899, based on his doctoral dissertation undertaken at Columbia University under the supervision of James Cattell, that voluntary movements are more accurate if performed more slowly, thus establishing the trade-off between speed and accuracy in their performance.[1] This speed-accuracy trade-off may perhaps apply to any task, and since speed is inversely proportional to time it may also be formulated as a time-accuarcy trade-off, longer times being required for greater accuracy.[2]

Woodworth finds a place in the history of psychology as the author of text-books, *Psychology: a study of mental life* (1921) and *Experimental psychology* (1938), and for his "S-O-R framework" (Stimulus-Organism-Response) for experimental research in psychology.[3] He taught at Columbia from 1903 for the rest of his long career, which included the Presidency of the American Psychological Association in 1914.

Little mentioned, but of potentially particular interest to British readers, is Woodworth's fellowship working with Charles Scott Sherrington (1857–1952) at the University of Liverpool, taken up in 1902. There are few accounts of the workings of Sherrington's laboratory during this phase of his career: he was in Liverpool as Holt Professor of Physiology between 1895 and 1913. This period notably encompassed Sherrington's Silliman Memorial Lectures at Yale in 1904 which were to become his seminal work, *The integrative action of the nervous system*, first published in 1906.

Woodworth did publish some autobiographical notes in 1932,[4] but sadly these say very little about his time in Liverpool, the only references to Sherrington being these:

The physiologists with whom I studied and taught were Bowditch and Porter of Harvard, Graham Lusk of New York, Schafer [*sic*] of Edinburgh, and Sherrington, then at Liverpool. My physiological studies were on the heart, stomach movements, carbohydrate metabolism, electrical conductivity of nerve, cerebral localization, and reflex action. (367).

At the beginning of 1903, then, I was Sherrington's assistant at Liverpool, and much minded to make my psychology contribute to a career in brain physiology, rather than vice versa. Sherrington, to whom I owe very much, was willing that I should remain with him and develop my experimental psychology and brain physiology together. Just at this point, Cattell called me back to Columbia ... (368).

Of course, Sherrington was still alive at the time Woodworth published these autobiographical notes, indeed he shared the Nobel Prize in that year (1932) with E.D. Adrian, so this might have inhibited Woodworth from saying more. At a distance of nearly 30 years, Woodworth may have forgotten much, or now considered this a minor interlude in his career, a temporary diversion into physiology from a path destined for psychology.

We would of course like to know more about the mechanics of their interactions in research, the precise work undertaken, the other workers in the laboratory. The only first-hand account of Sherrington's Liverpool laboratory of which I am currently aware is that contained in Harvey Cushing's letters describing what his biographer, John Fulton, calls "A month with Sherrington" (in fact, Cushing arrived in Liverpool on 7th July 1901, and departed in August, but Sherrington had left on 29th July).[5] Clearly this predates Woodworth's time in Liverpool, but he would have overlapped with William Warrington, who was worked with Sherrington (ca. 1899–1904);[6] did they cross paths, interact in any way?

Sherrington worked in the Thompson Yates and Johnston Laboratories at the University of Liverpool, which between 1898 and 1905 had its own house journal, initially called the *Thompson Yates Laboratories Report* and latterly (from 1903) the *Thompson Yates and Johnston Laboratories Report*. Woodworth appears in Volume 5 Part 1, published in 1903. Firstly he is amongst those, including Warrington, listed as having "assisted" the editors, Rubert Boyce and Sherrington (along with Annett, Grünbaum, Moore, Ross, and Hope). He also has a short paper on "The electrical conductivity of mammalian nerve" where his affiliation is given as "Senior demonstrator of physiology, and formerly G.W. Garrett Fellow in the University of Liverpool".[7] This work followed up the substantial study on the injury current of nerve which had been undertaken by J.S. Macdonald and reported in Volume 4 (1902) of the *Thompson Yates Laboratories Report* (pages 213–349). Sherrington was not mentioned in Woodworth's publication, and he did not appear in Volume 5 part 2 published in December 1903.

One paper, at least, emerged from Woodworth's collaboration with Sherrington (although it was not mentioned in Woodworth's autobiographical piece): "A pseudaffective reflex and its spinal path".[8] This work, examining mimetic movements in the decerebrate cat simulating expression of certain affective states, is mentioned by Sherrington in *The integrative action of the nervous system*.[9] It is also included in the bibliography of Sherrington's papers, prepared by Fulton, in Liddell's obituary notice of Sherrington, but there is no other mention of Woodworth therein.[10]

In his account of the "Sherrington School" of physiology, published over 50 years later, Derek Denny-Brown distinguished between those Sherrington "collaborated with" and the "many others [who] published work from his laboratory under his guidance"[11] (p. 543). Woodworth appears in the former category, Warrington in the latter, Cushing in neither. However, it seems that Cushing, unlike Woodworth, kept in touch with Sherrington by correspondence.[12]

Acknowledgement

Unpublished manuscript, early 2024.

References

1. Woodworth RS. Accuracy of voluntary movements. Psychol Rev. 1899; 3: 1–101.
2. Larner AJ. Performance-based cognitive screening instruments: an extended analysis of the time versus accuracy trade-off. Diagnostics (Basel). 2015; 5: 504–512.
3. Benjafield JG. *A history of psychology* (4th edition). Oxford: Oxford University Press, 2015:184–187.
4. Murchison C (ed.). *A history of psychology in autobiography. Volume II*. New York: Russell and Russell, 1932 [1961]: 359–380.
5. Fulton JB. *Harvey Cushing. A biography*. Springfield, Illinois: Charles C. Thomas, 1946: 195–200.
6. Larner AJ. William Barnett Warrington (1869–1919). In: Larner AJ. *Neuroliterature 2. Biography, semiology, miscellany. Further literary perspectives on disorders of the nervous system*. Gloucester: Choir Press, 2023: 125–137.
7. Woodworth RS. The electrical conductivity of mammalian nerve. Thompson Yates and Johnston Laboratories Report. 1903; 5: 61–66.
8. Woodworth RS, Sherrington CS. A pseudaffective reflex and its spinal path. J Physiol. 1904; 31: 234–243.
9. Sherrington CS. *The integrative action of the nervous system*. New Haven: Yale University Press 1906 [1926]: 251, 295.
10. Liddell EGT. Charles Scott Sherrington 1857–1952. Obit Not Fell R Soc. 1952; 8: 241–270.

11. Denny-Brown D. The Sherrington School of physiology. J Neurophysiol. 1957; 20: 543–548.

12. Louis ED. The Sherrington-Cushing connection: a bench to bedside collaboration at the dawn of the twentieth century. J Hist Neurosci. 2020; 29: 203–220.

Lionel Penrose (1898–1972): a neuro-cultural note

Lionel Sharples Penrose was a noted medical geneticist of the mid-twentieth century,[1] a winner of the prestigious Lasker Prize in 1960.

At a relatively early stage in his career, Penrose undertook a study of "mental defect", published in 1938 under the auspices of the Medical Research Council (MRC) as *MRC Special Report: No. 229. Clinical and genetic study of 1,280 cases of mental defect*. It is sometimes known as the "Colchester Survey" since this is where the research was undertaken. However, some subsequent confusion as to the exact location of Penrose's work may have arisen.

In her short story *Trespassing* (2011),[2] the author Margaret Drabble describes the:

> ... listed properties that had been purpose-built in the late nineteenth and early twentieth century as asylums and psychiatric institutions ... They had served their purpose, and the medical theory and practice had moved on, as had the language that described the one-time inmates. Now they stood empty ... sad monuments to the pioneering hopes and the sullen despairs of the past ... (85)

She gives an account of:

> ... looking for the once-celebrated hospital where Lionel Penrose had worked on the Down's syndrome chromosome ... Although large and in its day famous, it was exceptionally hard to locate ... the building called Severalls ... it had housed two thousand inmates and a large staff (85–86).

Severalls Hospital, Colchester, opened in 1913, was the Second Essex County Asylum.[3]

However, contrary to Drabble, this was not where Penrose worked: Diana Gittins's history of the hospital has no mention of him.[4]

Penrose was appointed as "Research Medical Officer" to the Royal Eastern Counties Institution, sometimes known as the Eastern Counties Asylum for Idiots and Imbeciles, in Colchester in 1931. This institution had previously been known as Essex Hall, and was a branch of the Royal Earlswood Asylum. The history of this institution began with the opening in April 1848 of Park House in Highgate, later called the National Asylum for Idiots, with further accommodation later opened at Essex Hall, Colchester. Subsequently a purpose-built asylum was constructed at Earlswood near Redhill in Surrey, opening in 1855. John Langdon Down (1828–1896), known to posterity for his description of "mongoloid idiots", was superintendent at Earlswood from 1858 to 1868.[5]

As a consequence of his studies at the Royal Eastern Counties Institution, Penrose rebutted Langdon Down's original suggestion of "mongoloid idiocy" based on a notion of "Mongoloid ancestry", suggesting that in its place the term "Down's syndrome" or "Down's anomaly" should be used. It was not until 1959 that Lejeune reported the chromosomal anomaly of trisomy 21 which was shown to be the genetic cause of most cases of Down's syndrome.

Another, perhaps more familiar, cultural influence of Penrose is the description of the Penrose stairs or steps,[6] published in 1958 with his son Roger (later a distinguished mathematician and winner of the Nobel Prize in Physics in 2020). This had been prompted by Roger's experience of seeing the works of M.C. Escher (1898–1972), to whom the impossible figure was then sent, and who used it in his celebrated drawing *Ascending and descending* of 1960.

References

1. Harris H. Lionel Sharples Penrose, 1898–1972. *Biogr Mem Fellows R Soc* 1973; 19: 521–561.
2. Drabble M. Trespassing. In: *The Guardian Review book of short stories.* London: Guardian, 2011: 83–96.
3. www.countyasylums.co.uk
4. Gittins D. *Madness in its place: narratives of Severalls Hospital, 1913–1997.* London: Routledge, 1998.
5. Wright D. *Mental disability in Victorian England. The Earlswood Asylum 1847–1901.* Oxford: Oxford University Press, 2001.
6. Penrose LS, Penrose R. Impossible objects: a special type of visual illusion. Br J Psychology 1958; 49: 31–33

T.P.S. Powell (1923–1996): a centenary appreciation

2023 marks the centenary of the birth of Thomas ("Tom") Powell. Although originally a clinician by training, he is best known for his neuroscientific studies on the anatomy of the mammalian cerebral cortex but he made many other contributions, including to the neuropathology of Alzheimer's disease [1,2]. Moreover, he is still fondly remembered as an inspirational teacher of basic neuroanatomy to generations of undergraduate medical students at Oxford University.

Thomas Philip Stroud Powell was born in South Wales, the son of a miner. After qualifying in medicine at Edinburgh University in 1945, he undertook clinical posts before joining the Cambridge University Anatomy Department in 1946 as a demonstrator to prepare for the Primary Fellowship of the Royal College of Surgeons (FRCS). Passing this examination, he continued his surgical training in Edinburgh (with Norman Dott) and at Hammersmith Hospital in London, becoming FRCS in 1950. In 1951 he won a Medical Research Council clinical research fellowship to study with the neurosurgeon Hugh Cairns (1896–1952) in Oxford, who sent him to pursue experimental studies in the laboratory of the anatomist Wilfrid Le Gros Clark (1895–1971). This resulted in Powell's first publication, in *Brain* [3], and set him on the pathway of a career exploring the functional connectivity of the brain, descriptive neuroanatomy winning out over a career in medicine. Nevertheless, he never forgot his clinical roots.

The technique of retrograde degeneration utilised in his first paper also informed a number of Powell's early studies of thalamocortical connections and septo-hippocampal pathways. In the mid-1950s a fruitful collaboration was begun with Maxwell Cowan (1931–2002) with whom he eventually co-authored over 30 papers between 1954 and 1967 [4]. These included examinations of the connections of the thalamus, hippocampus, fornix, mammillary bodies, amygdala, striatum, visual system, and olfactory system, using techniques of anterograde tracing and transneuronal cell degeneration, for example in the lateral geniculate nucleus. Later monocular deprivation (eye suture) studies in infant macaque monkeys showed profound atrophy of cells in the deafferented layers of this nucleus. Powell and his collaborators also used the Glees silver method to show orthograde degeneration of nerve fibres and later the more reliable Nauta technique.

An important interlude in this programme of neuroanatomical research at Oxford was Powell's visit to America between December 1956 and April 1958 on a Rockefeller Foundation Travelling Fellowship to Johns Hopkins Hospital in Baltimore USA where he worked with Vernon B. Mountcastle (1918–2015) [5]. This was shortly after the latter had established the columnar architecture of the somatosensory cortex. Together, Powell and Mountcastle published four papers in the *Bulletin of the Johns Hopkins Hospital* in 1959 [6]. In the words of David Hubel and Torsten Wiesel, who were later to adopt and adapt these techniques most successfully in their seminal studies of the visual cortex, Powell and Mountcastle devised "a method ... for studying cells separately or in small groups during long micro-electrode penetrations through nervous tissue. Responses are correlated with cell location by reconstructing the electrode tracks from histological material. These techniques have been applied to the somatic sensory cortex of the cat and monkey in a remarkable series of studies" [7].

Powell's most productive years were spent in Oxford in the 1960s and 1970s working with a succession of DPhil students. The techniques of electron microscopy were added to his previous light microscopy studies of thalamo-cortical connections. Many of his publications appeared in the *Philosophical Transactions of the Royal Society*, and his work culminated in election to the Fellowship of the Royal Society (FRS) in 1978, making him one of the very few individuals to be simultaneously both FRCS and FRS.

In the 1980s Powell increasingly pursued problems of more clinical relevance, perhaps reflecting his clinical origins. In particular, he was involved in studies of the brain in Alzheimer's disease (AD) in collaboration with, amongst others, RCA Pearson, Margaret Esiri, and Mike Sofroniew. A number of studies examined the cholinergic nuclei of the basal forebrain in the rat [8], the principal source of cholinergic input to the cortex, the loss of which in AD later provided the rationale for the first meaningful strategy for the treatment of AD. An examination of the distribution of neurofibrillary tangles and neuritic plaques in AD neocortex, specifically the severe involvement of association areas with the relative sparing of primary motor and sensory (somatosensory, visual, auditory) areas, led to the proposal of spread of pathological changes along interconnecting pathways, perhaps originating in the olfactory areas [9], a proposal predating the subsequent Braak classification of neurofibrillary change in AD brain. A subsequent quantitative study of neurofibrillary tangles and choline acetyltransferase activity in AD brains was adduced as support for the hypothesis of a spreading disease process, either anterograde or retrograde, along a sequence of cortico-cortical connections and/or between the neocortex and amygdala [10]. Further recognition of Powell's work came with the award of the Bristol-Myers prize (jointly) in 1989. He retired in 1990, his final publication appearing in 1991.

In addition to his research work, Powell made extensive contributions to the teaching of Oxford University medical students throughout his career, both within the Department of Human Anatomy and, from 1952, at St John's College where he was elected to a Fellowship in 1963. Subsequently he also gave tutorials at Trinity and Worcester Colleges. With his clinical background, he was well equipped to inculcate the key aspects of neuroanatomy to preclinical medical students.

Acknowledgement

I thank Dr Michael Mansfield for drawing my attention to Tom Powell, 25/03/2023. Unpublished manuscript, mid-2023.

References

1. Guillery RW (1997) Thomas Philip Stroud Powell. 13 July 1923 – 8 February 1996. Biogr Mems Fell R Soc 43:412–427
2. Jones EG (1999) Making brain connections: neuroanatomy and the work of TPS Powell, 1923–1996. Annu Rev Neurosci 22:49–103
3. Powell TPS (1952) Residual neurons in the human thalamus following hemidecortication. Brain 75:57–84
4. Raisman G (2008) William Maxwell Cowan. 27 September 1931 – 30 June 2002. Biogr Mems Fell R Soc 54:117–136
5. Cambiaghi M (2020) Vernon B. Mountcastle (1918–2015). J Neurol 267:298–299
6. Powell TP, Mountcastle VB (1959) Some aspects of the functional organization of the cortex of the postcentral gyrus of the monkey: a correlation of findings obtained in a single unit analysis with cytoarchitecture. Bull Johns Hopkins Hosp 105:133–162
7. Hubel DH, Wiesel TN (1962) Receptive fields, binocular interaction and functional architecture in the cat's visual cortex. J Physiol 160:106–154
8. Sofroniew MV, Esiri MM, Powell TP (1987) The cholinergic nuclei of the basal forebrain of the rat: normal structure, development and experimentally induced degeneration. Brain Res 411:310–331
9. Pearson RC, Esiri MM, Hiorns RW, Wilcock GK, Powell TP (1985) Anatomical correlates of the distribution of the pathological changes in the neocortex in Alzheimer disease. Proc Natl Acad Sci USA 82:4531–4534
10. Esiri MM, Pearson RC, Steele JE, Bowen DM, Powell TP (1990) A quantitative study of the neurofibrillary tangles and the choline acetyltransferase activity in the cerebral cortex and the amygdala in Alzheimer's disease. J Neurol Neurosurg Psychiatry 53:161–165

David Marsden (1938–1998): contributions to cognitive neurology

For neurologists of a certain age, it may come as something of a surprise, if not a shock, to realise that 2023 will mark a quarter of a century since the untimely death of Professor CD Marsden. In part this surprise may be related to the fact that publications bearing the Marsden imprimatur continued to appear long after his death, culminating in the eponymous *Marsden's Book of Movement Disorders*[1] which, though contemplated many years earlier, did not make its first appearance until late 2011/early 2012.

David Marsden is rightly known for his influential contributions, clinical, neuroscientific and administrative, to the field of movement disorders (one of his obituaries described him as "Master of Movement"), but his interests were not limited by this specialisation. As a consequence of his many collaborations, he was an author on many papers pertaining to cognitive function and its disorders, either directly or indirectly. A brief review of some of these is given here, restricted to clinical reports, in part to commemorate but also to illustrate the breadth of Marsden's contributions. It should be emphasized that this review does not claim to be exhaustive, and is given from the perspective of an outsider, not someone who ever worked in any capacity for Professor Marsden. An account from those who knew and worked with him is published,[2] which briefly alludes to his studies of cognitive deficits in parkinsonian disorders (p.212).

1/ Dementia

"Presenile" dementia
One of Marsden's earliest publications, dating from 1972, was based on work undertaken as, according the paper in the *BMJ*, Senior Registrar at Queen Square, on the subject of (so called) "presenile" dementia.[3] Working with Michael Harrison (d. 2019), a retrospective study of more than 100 patients was presented, in whom intellectual impairment was confirmed in 84 and a "final" diagnosis established in 36. Aside from "cerebral atrophy of unknown cause" (n = 48), many presumed to have Alzheimer's disease or Pick's disease, intracranial space-occupying mass lesion and arteriosclerotic dementia were the next most common diagnoses (both n = 8). Of the 22 patients classified with no or uncertain dementia, depression was the most common diagnosis. This study predated the availability of CT brain scanning; lumbar air encephalography was the most sophisticated neuroimaging investigation

available. Moreover, the initial paper gave neither a definition of "presenile" nor details of the age of the patients investigated; the latter information emerged in a subsequent letter (age range 34–78, mean 61 years).[4]

"Senile" dementia

Patients with "senile" dementia, meaning onset over 65 years of age, formed one group, along with Parkinson's disease and "cerebral arteriosclerosis," in a 1974 study examining clinical features and response to levodopa. Evidently, the dementia patients were in the severe stage of disease, frequently unable to walk or stand; half of them reportedly had "whole body akinesia". Predictably, they did not respond to levodopa, and indeed as a group they showed deterioration in rigidity when treated.[5]

Cortical versus subcortical dementia

Distinction between dementia ascribed respectively to cortical or subcortical pathology enjoyed something of a vogue in the 1980s and 1990s. So called cortical dementia was typified by the classical syndromes of amnesia, aphasia, and agnosia, whereas so called subcortical dementia, a terminology first used in the context of progressive supranuclear palsy, was typified by cognitive slowing, sometimes with apathy and depression. Brown and Marsden's review of these concepts, in the context of Alzheimer's disease, Parkinson's disease and Huntington's disease, found more overlap than separation in deficits between the patient groups, hence casting doubt on the functional independence of these two broad diagnostic categories.[6]

Alzheimer's disease

Alzheimer's disease (AD) was not an area of particular clinical interest for Marsden but was encountered from time to time in the context of concurrent movement disorder. He was one of the authors on papers describing the alien hand sign[7] and frontal gait impairment[8] in patients found to have underlying Alzheimer's disease pathology. In the first of these reports, the patient had a clinical diagnosis of corticobasal degeneration prior to the availability of neuropathological findings[7] (hence what might now be termed corticobasal syndrome). In the second paper, the one patient in whom neuropathology was available had histological features of corticobasal degeneration as well as AD pathology, the latter most evident in the occipital cortex with relative sparing of the hippocampus.[8] Alzheimer-type changes were also observed along with cerebrovascular pathology in a patient presenting with a late onset generalised chorea.[9]

A group of patients with "probable dementia of Alzheimer type" was investigated with tests of visual memory and tests sensitive to frontal lobe dysfunction as a comparator group for patients with Huntington's disease (vide infra) matched for "level of dementia," as defined by Mini-Mental State Examination (MMSE) score. The AD patients were found to be more impaired on tests of recall but superior on the tests sensitive to frontal lobe dysfunction than the Huntington's disease patients.[10]

2/ Cognitive features of movement disorders

It is perhaps easy to forget from our vantage point that the differentiation of Parkinson's disease from other parkinsonian disorders, sometimes labelled as "atypical parkinsonism" or "Parkinson's plus," was not so clear cut in the late 1970s/early 1980s, when Marsden and his colleagues began publishing on the subject, than is now the case. Certainly one of debts we owe to them relates to the empirical studies which clarified this differential, including cognitive features.

Parkinson's disease
Whilst Charcot, unlike James Parkinson, had recognised that cognitive impairment could be a feature of the disorder upon which he had bestowed the eponymous label of Parkinson's disease (PD), relatively little attention was paid to this aspect of PD until the 1970s and 1980s. Marsden's engagement with the cognitive consequences of PD was evident in a *Lancet* review co-authored with Richard Brown published in 1984 examining dementia in PD.[11] A downward revision of the frequency of dementia in PD from 1 in 3 to a more conservative 1 in 5 was suggested, in part due to diagnostic errors in distinguishing PD from other akinetic-rigid syndromes. This conclusion was based on the data then available, whereas subsequent studies have suggested a much higher cumulative frequency of cognitive impairment in PD.

As for the specific cognitive features encountered in PD, Marsden was involved in a number of studies examining these, dating back to the early 1970s.[5] Many years later, the cognitive deficits in PD were characterized in comparison to other parkinsonian syndromes, finding slowing in initial thinking time (bradyphrenia) and impairments on tests of frontal lobe function.[12]

Progressive supranuclear palsy
In the study comparing various parkinsonian syndromes, patients with progressive supranuclear palsy (PSP) were shown to have cognitive deficits on tests of frontal lobe function, like PD patients, but the greatest deficit in attentional set shifting was found in PSP patients.[12]

Multiple system atrophy

Multiple system atrophy (MSA) was generally thought to be free from cognitive dysfunction prior to a report on a "distinctive pattern" of cognitive deficits in MSA of striato-nigral predominance (MSA-P) by Marsden and his colleagues. This showed a prominent frontal-lobe-like component,[13] later confirmed in a larger study.[12]

Corticobasal degeneration

Marsden and his colleagues were some of the first to undertake systematic studies of patients with corticobasal degeneration (CBD). Understandably this was largely from the perspective of the movement disorders rather than the cognitive features, for example they reported that "Cognitive changes are unusual early in the disease, the intellect being preserved".[14] Although noting the emergence of aphasia in some patients, there was no apparent awareness of non-fluent aphasic presentations of CBD with subsequent emergence of the typical motor features of CBD, as noted by later authors.

Huntington's disease

The cognitive features of Huntington's disease (HD) were compared to those in AD patients and shown to be distinct, with poorer performance on tests examining frontal lobe function, suggestive of a frontostriatial pattern of dysfunction.[10]

3/ Other contributions

Apraxia

The nature of apraxia, and the possible role(s) of the basal ganglia in its pathogenesis, was one of Marsden's enduring interests.[15] Apraxia was examined in various parkinsonian patient groups. In CBD severe ideomotor and ideational apraxia was found to correlate with global cognitive impairment.[16] Apraxia was also observed in PSP (three-quarters of patients) and PD (about one quarter of patients) but was not seen in MSA and neuroleptic-induced parkinsonism. Ideomotor apraxia in PSP correlated with cognitive deficit (MMSE scores) and in PD with deficits in frontal lobe related tasks.[17]

Amnesia

Early in his clinical career (1974), Marsden was one of the authors on a classic paper showing that posterior cerebral artery occlusion may be a cause of acute onset of amnesia, so called "amnesic stroke," in association with unilateral or bilateral visual field defects. Although diagnosis of these patients was based on clinical evaluation alone,[18] the inferences were amply confirmed by later neuroimaging studies. Occasional cases of amnesic stroke are still reported, some with a phenotype apparently indistinguishable from transient global amnesia.

Discussion

Like one of his illustrious predecessors at Queen Square, William Gowers (1845–1915),[19] David Marsden made contributions in the field of cognitive disorders, incidental to his major clinical interests. Since disorders of cognition occur not only in isolation but also as components of more widespread diseases of the nervous system, they may be encountered by clinicians with interests in areas other than cognitive function. The specific pattern of cognitive deficits may be helpful in differential diagnosis. The groundwork of David Marsden and his colleagues facilitated this clinical understanding.

Acknowledgement

Adapted from: Larner AJ. David Marsden (1938–1998): contributions to cognitive neurology. *Adv Clin Neurosci Rehabil* 2023;22(1):22–23.

References

1. Donaldson I, Marsden CD, Schneider SA, Bhatia KP. *Marsden's Book of Movement Disorders.* Oxford: Oxford University Press, 2012

2. Quinn N, Rothwell J, Jenner P. *Charles David Marsden. 15 April 1938 – 29 September 1998.* Biogr Mems Fell R Soc 2012;58:203–228.

3. Marsden CD, Harrison MJG. *Outcome of investigation of patients with presenile dementia.* BMJ 1972;2(5808):249–252.

4. Marsden CD, Harrison MJG. *Presenile dementia.* BMJ 1972;3(5817):50–51.

5. Parkes JD, Marsden CD, Rees JE, et al. *Parkinson's disease, cerebral arteriosclerosis, and senile dementia. Clinical features and response to levodopa.* Q J Med 1974;43:49–61.

6. Brown RG, Marsden CD. *"Subcortical dementia": the neuropsychological evidence.* Neuroscience 1988;25:363–387.

7. Ball JA, Lantos PL, Jackson M, Marsden CD, Scadding JW, Rossor MN. *Alien hand sign in association with Alzheimer's histopathology.* J Neurol Neurosurg Psychiatry 1993;56:1020–1023.

8. Rossor MN, Tyrrell PJ, Warrington EK, Thompson PD, Marsden CD, Lantos P. *Progressive frontal gait disturbance with atypical Alzheimer's disease and corticobasal degeneration.* J Neurol Neurosurg Psychiatry 1999;67:345–352.

9. Bhatia KP, Lera G, Luthert PJ, Marsden CD. *Vascular chorea: case report with pathology.* Mov Disord 1994;9:447–50.

10. Lange KW, Sahakian BJ, Quinn NP, Marsden CD, Robbins TW. *Comparison*

of executive and visuospatial memory function in Huntington's disease and dementia of Alzheimer type matched for degree of dementia. J Neurol Neurosurg Psychiatry 1995;58:598–606.

11. Brown RG, Marsden CD. *How common is dementia in Parkinson's disease?* Lancet 1984;2(8414):1262–1265.

12. Robbins TW, James M, Owen AM, Lange KW, Lees AJ, Leigh PN, Marsden CD, Quinn NP, Summers BA. *Cognitive deficits in progressive supranuclear palsy, Parkinson's disease, and multiple system atrophy in tests sensitive to frontal lobe dysfunction.* J Neurol Neurosurg Psychiatry 1994;57:79–88.

13. Robbins TW, James M, Lange KW, Owen AM, Quinn NP, Marsden CD. *Cognitive performance in multiple system atrophy.* Brain 1992;115:271–291.

14. Thompson PD, Marsden CD. *Corticobasal degeneration.* In: Rossor MN (ed.). *Unusual dementias.* London: Bailliere Tindall, 1992:677–686.

15. Pramstaller PP, Marsden CD. *The basal ganglia and apraxia.* Brain 1996;119:319–340.

16. Leiguarda RC, Lees AJ, Merello M, Starkstein S, Marsden CD. *The nature of apraxia in corticobasal degeneration.* J Neurol Neurosurg Psychiatry 1994;57:455–459.

17. Leiguarda RC, Pramstaller PP, Merello M, Starkstein S, Lees AJ, Marsden CD. *Apraxia in Parkinson's disease, progressive supranuclear palsy, multiple system atrophy and neuroleptic-induced parkinsonism.* Brain 1997;120:75–90.

18. Benson DF, Marsden CD, Meadows JC. *The amnesic syndrome of posterior cerebral artery occlusion.* Acta Neurol Scand 1974;50:133–145.

19. Larner AJ. *Sir William Gowers (1845–1915): a centenary celebration, with an examination of his comments on cognitive dysfunction.* Adv Clin Neurosci Rehabil 2015;15(1):16–17.

Semiology

Dermo-optical perception vs. colour-touch synaesthesia: further thoughts

In the seventeenth century, Robert Burton stated that "A blind man cannot judge of colours",[1] but it is possible that there may be exceptions!

An apparently fanciful account of "a Man born blind, who has several Apprentices in his own Condition: Their Employment was to mix Colours for Painters, which their master taught them to distinguish by feeling and smelling" appeared in Swift's *Gulliver's Travels* of 1726. This may have been based, at least in part, on an account by Robert Boyle in *Experiments and Considerations Touching Colours. First occasionally Written, among some other Essays, to a Friend; and now suffer'd to come abroad as the Beginning of an Experimental History of Colours*, published in 1664, which documented that "there lived one at some miles distance from Maestricht, who could distinguish Colours by the Touch".

It has been suggested that this individual, John Vermaasen, who "when he was but two years Old, he had the Small Pox, which rendred [*sic*] him absolutely Blind", may have had a synaesthetic condition in which tactile sensation is perceived as colour.[2] This formulation of colour-touch or colour-tactile synaesthesia was subsequently challenged (without the opportunity for reply) by Brugger and Weiss, who suggested that Boyle's account is in fact an example of dermo-optical perception, or fingertip sight.[3]

Occasional individuals have been described over the years who can apparently read print, describe pictures, and recognise colours purely by way of touch. One such example, recounted by James Crichton-Browne (1840–1938), was "blind Alick of Stirling" who "became blind in infancy". According to his grandmother, who told Crichton-Browne the story:

> She remembered a test applied to him, when a number of soldiers belonging to her husband's regiment and a number of civilians were drawn up in line in no definite order, while Alick walked along the line touching with his forefinger the coat of each as he passed. In every instance he distinguished the soldier from the civilian. He made no mistake and it seemed certain that at any rate he was able to recognise a material having a scarlet colour.
>
> It was alleged that he acquired his power of distinguishing colours by manipulating the dresses of his schoolfellows when they tried to deceive him as to their identity by using feigned voices. It was chiefly in distinguishing the colours of woollen fabrics that he excelled; with silks and cottons he had difficulties.[4]

Of course, it is possible that the discrimination of soldier from civilian could have been by touch alone (scarlet/not scarlet) based on the material of the soldiers' regimentals (or even on other sensory cues, such as smell). For Vermassen "all the difference was more or less Asperity", his account being that:

> Black and White are the most asperous or unequal of all Colours, and so like, that 'tis very hard to distinguish them, but Black is the most Rough of the two, Green is next in Asperity, Gray next to Green in Asperity, Yellow is the fifth in degree of Asperity, Red and Blew [*sic*] are so like, that they are as hard to distinguish as Black and White, but Red is somewhat more Asperous than Blew, so that Red has the sixth place, and Blew the seventh in Asperity.

There is also a hint of colours having a tactile quality, including roughness, in Luria's classic account of his synaesthetic mnemonist "S", Shereshevsky (e.g. "rough colours").[5] Blind patients "seeing" Braille characters as coloured dots when they were touched has also been reported.[6] This visual/tactile linkage may have been anticipated by Hughlings Jackson: speaking of the ocular phenomena of migraine, he noted that "the zigzag or fortification outline [visual aura] implies excitation of motor elements; of those I suppose which serve in giving us ideas (symbolically of tactual ideas) of roughness (minute shapes), and which are so immediately, inevitably, and deeply organised with the corresponding retinal impressions that roughness and colour seem to be one sensation."[7]

Is this faculty, of sensing colours by touch, apparent rather than genuine? In the 18th century, Samuel Johnson denied the possibility, based on the statement of Nicholas Saunderson, Lucasian Professor of Mathematics at the University of Cambridge who, blinded by smallpox at the age of twelve months, had attempted the feat without success.[8] Nevertheless, could it be that, in response to sensory deprivation such as blindness, tactile sense is augmented to such an extent (hyperpilaphesie) that in some individuals it permits colour discrimination? It would be interesting to test congenitally blind individuals, with no colour concept, with different coloured objects of identical material to see if any difference was sensed (note that several of the reported cases – Vermassen, Alick – became blind at a young age).

To my knowledge, it remains the case that no studies using modern neuroscientific investigations have been reported in individuals claiming to have dermo-optical perception, whereas cases of colour-touch or colour-tactile synaesthesia, although very uncommon, have been studied.[9] This case (patient EB) showed that tactile qualities such as smoothness and roughness were systematically related to the luminance and chroma of associated colours, thus permitting the patient to develop an implicit rule system for recognition. Hence it may be that visual information can be transmitted through haptic channels, as suggested by some of the historical case reports.

Acknowledgement

Unpublished manuscript, early 2024.

References

1. Gowland A (ed.). *Robert Burton. The anatomy of melancholy.* London: Penguin Classics, 2021:441.
2. Larner AJ. A possible account of synaesthesia dating from the seventeenth century. *J Hist Neurosci* 2006;15:245–249. (Reprinted with adaptations in: Larner AJ. *Neuroliterature: Patients, doctors, diseases. Literary perspectives on disorders of the nervous system.* Gloucester: Choir Press, 2019:177–182.)
3. Brugger P, Weiss PH. Dermo-optical perception: the non-synesthetic "palpability of colors" a comment on Larner (2006). *J Hist Neurosci* 2008;17:253–255.
4. Crichton-Browne J. *Victorian jottings from an old commonplace book.* London: Etchells and Macdonald, 1926:11–12.
5. Luria AR. *The mind of a mnemonist. A little book about a vast memory.* New York: Basic Books, 1968:81,83.
6. Cytowic RE, Eagleman DM. *Wednesday is indigo blue. Discovering the brain of synesthesia.* Cambridge: MIT Press, 2011:44–45.
7. Jackson JH. On epilepsies and on the after effects of epileptic discharges (Todd and Robertson's hypothesis). *West Riding Lunatic Asylum Medical Reports* 1876; 6: 266–309 [at 275].
8. Brewer FA. Samuel Johnson on dermo-optical perception. *Science* 1966;152:592.
9. Simner J, Ludwig VU. The color of touch: a case of tactile-visual synaesthesia. *Neurocase* 2012;18:167–180.

Eponymous neurological syndromes and signs: literary and historical

Neurologists are familiar with many eponyms that populate their discipline. These include diseases (e.g. Alzheimer, Parkinson, Pick, Huntington, Wilson) and syndromes (e.g Jacksonian epilepsy) and neurological signs (e.g. Babinski, Gowers, Tinel, Argyll Robertson, Todd) named for the individual who first described or brought to general attention the syndrome or sign.[1] Naturally enough, many neurologists are interested in the clinicians thus commemorated, wish to know more about their lives and works, and may feel an affinity with their clinical endeavours.

It is recognised that such eponyms have their shortcomings. Individuals so commemorated may have an unsavoury or even criminal past (e.g. clinicians associated with the Nazi regime: Asperger, Spatz), or may not have been the first to describe the illness or sign for which they are named. Moreover, medical advances more often depend on collaborative work, discussion, and consensus rather than on isolated individuals. Accordingly, some recommend that eponyms be abandoned.[2,3]

Another category of eponyms, to be explored briefly here, derives from literary characters or places or from non-medical historical individuals after whom diseases and signs are named. I suspect that these are fewer than those named for clinicians. The following listing does not claim to be exhaustive.

1. Eponymous neurological syndromes and signs based on literary characters/places

Diseases/Syndromes

Perhaps unsurprisingly, many of the entries in this category relate to classic literary works, such as those by Shakespeare, Cervantes, Dickens, and Lewis Carroll.

Othello syndrome

Named for Shakespeare's Othello, this is a syndrome of pathological, morbid, or delusional jealousy revolving around a belief in a partner's infidelity without legitimate proof.[4]

Ophelia syndrome
Named for Shakespeare's Ophelia from *Hamlet*, this describes memory loss in patients with Hodgkin's disease.[5] This is now recognised to be an autoimmune limbic encephalitis associated with mGluR5 antibodies.

Don Quixote syndrome
Named for Cervantes' character, this has been suggested to describe a transformation from reading fictional literature[6] or a delusion of greatness or of noble intent.[7]

Rip van Winkle syndrome (or disease)
Named after Washington Irving's character Rip van Winkle who falls asleep for twenty years, this name has come to be used to describe Kleine-Levin syndrome, a rare disorder usually afflicting teenage boys and characterised by hypersomnolence, hyperphagia, and sometimes hypersexuality.

Pickwickian syndrome
The character of Joe the fat boy in Dickens's *Posthumous papers of the Pickwick Club* is described as obese, ruddy, somnolent, and has dropsy, a constellation of symptoms which has been retrospectively identified with obstructive sleep apnoea.

Miss Havisham syndrome
This character from Dickens's *Great Expectations* adopts a reclusive lifestyle, attempting to make time stand still, after a major emotional shock. Critchley thought this merited an eponymous syndrome.[8]

Alice in Wonderland syndrome
Named after Lewis Carroll's character, Alice in Wonderland syndrome encompasses a large variety of perceptual distortions, both visual (metamorphopsia) and somaesthetic. Classification dependent on the nature of the distortions (A = somaesthetic; B = visual; C = both).[9]

Mad Hatter syndrome (or disease)
Mad Hatter's disease has been used as a synonym for mercury poisoning, or erethism, because of the use of mercury in the felt hat industry. Lewis Carroll's character, however eccentric, has none of the features of mercury poisoning.

Godot syndrome

Samuel Beckett's play *Waiting for Godot* is perhaps one of the most celebrated plays of the 20th century, spawning the use of "Godot syndrome" to describe anxiety for a forthcoming event (that may not happen).

"Render's syndrome"

Ursula Le Guin's account of "Render's syndrome" in her short story *Vaster than empires and more slow* takes its name from a character in a novel, *The Dream Master*, by Roger Zelazny, denoting supernormal empathic capacity.[10]

Neurological signs

Lilliput sight, Lilliputian hallucinations

Following Jonathan Swift's *Gulliver's Travels* (1726), these terms refer respectively to an illusory phenomenon in which the size of a normally recognized object is underestimated (micropsia) and seeing tiny people.

Malapropisms/Archie Bunker "syndrome"

Mrs Malaprop is a character in R.B. Sheridan's play *The Rivals* (1775) who misuses language to unintended comic effect, a trait shared (apparently) with Archie Bunker is the 1970s US television sitcom *All in the Family*.[11]

Popeye arms

Wasting of biceps and triceps with preserved deltoid and forearm muscles in facioscapulohumeral dystrophy has been likened to the appearances of the upper limbs in the cartoon character Popeye the Sailor.

Fonzarelli sign

Focal thumb dystonia producing a tonic "thumbs-up" gesture has been named after the character of Arthur ("Fonzie") Fonzarelli, played by Henry Winkler in the US TV sitcom *Happy Days*.[12]

2. Eponymous neurological syndromes and signs based on historical figures

Diseases/Syndromes
St Vitus' dance

St Vitus (possibly 3rd century CE) was a martyr whose feast day involved dancing, hence the name "St Vitus dance" became associated with the movement disorder also known as Sydenham's chorea.

Brueghel syndrome (sometimes spelled Breughel)

Brueghel syndrome is a dystonia of the motor trigeminal nerve causing gaping or involuntary opening of the mouth, so named after the painting by Pieter Brueghel the Elder (*ca.* 1525–1569).[13]

Diogenes syndrome

A syndrome characterised by self-neglect, domestic squalor, hoarding behaviour, and social withdrawal with refusal of external help, referring to Diogenes of Sinope (*ca.* 412–323 BC) who was noted for his austere asceticism and self-sufficiency and his disregard for domestic comforts.[14]

Fregoli delusion

This delusional disorder, charcaterised by misidnentification of a familiar person in other people, even though they bear no resemblance, is named for the Italian actor Leopoldo Fregoli (1867–1936) who was noted as a mimic.

Mona Lisa syndrome

The so-called enigmatic smile of the Mona Lisa (Lisa del Giocondo) as painted by Leonardo da Vinci has been suggested (by an otorhinolaryngologist) to depict synkinetic facial muscle contracture as a consequence of Bell's palsy.[15] Presumably she was unfortunate enough to have this affliction bilaterally?

Phineas Gage syndrome

A change in behaviour and social interactions as a consequence of frontal lobe injury, as described in Phineas Gage (1823–1860) following his accident in 1848 in which a tamping iron was blasted through his brain.

Lou Gehrig's disease

Lou Gehrig (1903–1941) was a baseball player with the New York Yankees who developed motor neurone disease around 1939, subsequently known in the United States as "Lou Gehrig's disease".

Neurological signs

Groucho Marx sign

Rapid repetitive wrinkling of the forehead, a trademark of Groucho Marx (1890–1977). May be used as a test of frontalis function.

Lazarus sign, Lazarus movements
Named after the individual raised from the dead by Christ, this refers to a spinal reflex occurring in brain death characterised by elbow flexion, shoulder adduction, lifting of the arms, and dystonic posturing of the hands.

Proust phenomenon
Proust phenomenon, after the writer Marcel Proust (1871–1922), also known as Petit madeleines phenomenon, refers to the triggering of specific authobiographical memories by particular odours,

Spoonerisms
The Reverend W.A. Spooner (1844–1930), sometime Warden of New College Oxford, was noted for a speech production disorder characterised by the transposition of consonants.

Discussion
Why are eponyms so common in clinical medicine? Do they relate solely to the clarity of description? To the desire to claim (rather than assign) priority? To the acknoweledgement of archetype? To the ease of relating to personal names rather than to purely descriptive titles? Any, all, or none of the above?

Acknowledgement

Unpublished manuscript, 2023–2024.

References

1. Larner AJ. *A dictionary of neurological signs* (4th edition). London: Springer, 2016.
2. Woywodt A, Matteson E. Should eponyms be abandoned? Yes. *BMJ* 2007;335:424.
3. Whitworth JA. Should eponyms be abandoned? No. *BMJ* 2007;335:425.
4. Todd J, Dewhurst K. The Othello syndrome: a study in the psychopathology of sexual jealousy. *J Nerv Ment Dis* 1955;122:367–74.
5. Carr I. The Ophelia syndrome: memory loss in Hodgkin's disease. *Lancet* 1982;1:844–5.
6. Iniesta I. Literature and epilepsy. *Medical Historian (Bulletin of Liverpool Medical History Society)* 2008–2009;20:31–53 [at 51].
7. Palma J-A, Palma F. Neurology and Don Quixote. *Eur Neurol* 2012;68:247–57.
8. Critchley M. *The divine banquet of the brain and other essays*. New York: Raven Press, 1979:136–140.

9. Blom JD. *Alice in Wonderland syndrome.* London: Springer, 2020.
10. Larner AJ. "Neurological literature": Render's syndrome. *Advances in Clinical Neuroscience & Rehabilitation* 2018;18(1):21.
11. Mendez MF. Malapropisms, or the "Archie Bunker syndrome," and frontotemporal dementia. *J Neuropsychiatry Clin Neurosci* 2011;23(4):E3.
12. Turner MR, Matthews L, Ebers GC. Teaching video NeuroImage: the "Fonzarelli" sign: focal thumb dystonia as an early manifestation of Parkinson's disease. *Neurology* 2008;71:e11.
13. Gilbert GJ. Brueghel syndrome: its distinction from Meige syndrome. *Neurology* 1996;46:1767–9.
14. Clarke ANG, Manikar GO, Gray I. Diogenes syndrome. A clinical study of gross neglect in old age. *Lancet* 1975;i:366–8.
15. Adour KK. Mona Lisa syndrome: solving the enigma of the Gioconda smile. *Ann Otol Rhinol Laryngol* 1989;98:196–9.

False localising signs: a topographical anatomy

Over one hundred and twenty years ago, Dr James Collier (1870–1935) published a paper in *Brain* entitled "The false localising signs of intracranial tumour". Based on his experience of 161 clinically and pathologically examined cases of intracranial tumour seen at the National Hospital, Queen Square, London, he observed false localising signs in 20 (12.4%).[1] The term was coined to indicate clinically observed signs that violated the expected clinico-anatomical concordance on which clinical examination is predicated.[2]

Since 1904, many examples of false localising signs have been described. They may occur in the clinical context of raised intracranial pressure (RICP) which is symptomatic of intracranial pathology (tumour, haematoma, abscess) or idiopathic (idiopathic intracranial hypertension: IIH), and with spinal cord lesions. Associated lesions may be intra- or extraparenchymal. The course of the associated disease may be acute (cerebral haematoma) or chronic (IIH, tumour).[3]

The pathogenesis of false localising signs remains uncertain, but their importance from a clinical standpoint is not in doubt, since they may lead to inappropriate imaging and even interventions on the wrong side (although the risk of such errors of commission is less now that neuroimaging is widely available). This article gives a brief topographical overview of false-localising signs. It does not claim to be exhaustive.

Brain: Motor system

False localising hemiparesis: Kernohan's notch syndrome
A supratentorial lesion, such as acute subdural haemaotoma, may cause transtentorial herniation of the temporal lobe, with compression of the ipsilateral cerebral peduncle against the tentorial edge; since this is above the pyramidal decussation a contralateral hemiparesis results. Occasionally, however, the hemiparesis may be ipsilateral to the lesion, and hence false localising; this occurs when the contralateral cerebral peduncle is compressed by the free edge of the tentorium. This is the Kernohan-Woltman notch phenomenon, or Kernohan's notch syndrome, first described in 1929,[4] also termed hemibrachiocrural syndrome. There may be concurrent homolateral third nerve palsy, ipsilateral to the causative lesion.[5] A literature review found most cases to be secondary to intracranial bleeds.[6]

False localising cerebellar syndrome

Frontocerebellar pathway damage, for example as a result of infarction in the territory of the anterior cerebral artery, may result in incoordination of the contralateral limbs, mimicking cerebellar dysfunction. Suboccipital exploration to search for cerebellar tumours based on these clinical findings was known to occur before the advent of brain imaging.[7]

False localising diaphragm paralysis due to brainstem compression

Hemidiaphragmatic paralysis with ipsilateral brainstem (medullary) compression by an aberrant vertebral artery has been described, in the absence of pathology localised to the C3–C5 segments of the spinal cord where phrenic motor neurones originate, hence a false-localizing sign.[8]

Brain: Sensory system

False localising sensory loss

Lateral medullary infarction typically causes, amongst other symptoms and signs, a crossed sensory pattern of loss, with contralateral hypoalgesia and thermoanaesthesia of the body (due to spinothalamic tract involvement) and ipsilateral facial hypoalgesia and thermoanaesthesia (due to trigeminal spinal nucleus and tract involvement). A case in which lateral medullary infarction was associated with isolated contralateral spinothalamic loss below the thoracic level, and hence false localising, has been reported.[9]

Brain: Cranial nerves

Oculomotor nerve (III)

Unilateral fixed dilated pupil (Hutchinson's pupil) may occur with an ipsilateral intracranial lesion such as an intracerebral haemorrhage, due to transtentorial herniation of the brain compressing the oculomotor nerve against the free edge of the tentorium. Because of the fascicluar organisation of fibres within the oculomotor nerve, the externally placed pupillomotor fibres are most vulnerable. Very occasionally, a fixed dilated pupil may occur contralateral to intracranial pathology, and hence false localising.[10] The exact mechanism for this clinical observation is not currently known.

Divisional third nerve palsy is usually associated with lesions at the superior orbital fissure or anterior cavernous sinus, where the superior division of the oculomotor nerve passes to the superior rectus and levator palpabrae, and the inferior division to the medial and inferior recti and inferior oblique muscles. Divisional third nerve palsies may sometimes occur with more proximal lesions, presumably as a consequence of the topographic arrangement of the fascicles within the nerve, for example with intrinsic brainstem disease (*e.g.* stroke)[11] or with pathology in the subarachnoid space where the nerve rootlets emerge from the brainstem (*e.g.* malignant infiltration).[12]

False localising third nerve palsy has occasionally been described in the context of IIH.[13]

Trochlear nerve (IV)
False localising fourth nerve palsy, causing diplopia on downward and inward gaze, has occasionally been described in the context of IIH.[14,15]

Trigeminal nerve (V)
Trigeminal nerve hypofunction (trigeminal sensory neuropathy) or hyperfunction (trigeminal neuralgia) may on occasion be false localising, for example in association with IIH,[16] or with contralateral pathology, often a tumour.[17] For example, trigeminal neuralgia has been associated with a contralateral chronic calcified subdural haematoma which caused rotational displacement of the pons, with resolution after removal of the haematoma.[18]

Abducens nerve (VI)
Sixth nerve palsies are the most common false localising sign of raised intracranial pressure. In one series of 101 cases of IIH, 14 cases were noted, 11 unilateral and 3 bilateral.[19] Stretching of the nerve in its long intracranial course or compression against the petrous ligament or ridge of the petrous temporal bone have been suggested as mechanisms for false localising sixth nerve palsy.[3]

Facial nerve (VII)
Lower motor neurone type facial weakness has been described in the context of IIH,[20] sometimes occurring bilaterally to cause facial diplegia,[21] usually with concurrent sixth nerve palsy (unilateral or bilateral).

Hemifacial spasm has rarely been described with contralateral posterior fossa lesions.[17]

Vestibulocochlear nerve (VIII)
Hearing loss has on occasion been reported as a complication of IIH,[22] although the commonest otological complication of IIH is tinnitus.[19]

Multiple and lower cranial nerve involvement
Concurrent false localising involvement of multiple cranial nerves has been noted on occasion, for example trigeminal, abducens and facial nerves with a contralateral acoustic neuroma,[23] and trigeminal, glossopharyngeal and vagus nerves with a contralateral laterally-placed posterior fossa meningioma.[24]

Impaired motor function of lower cranial nerves (V, VII, X, XI, XII) with unilateral cortical cerebrovascular lesions has also been reported.[25]

Spinal cord and roots

Foramen magnum/upper cervical cord

Paraesthesia in the hands with intrinsic hand muscle wasting and distal upper limb areflexia, with or without long tract signs, suggestive of a lower cervical myelopathy may occur with lesions at the foramen magnum or upper cervical cord ("remote atrophy").[26]

Lower cervical/upper thoracic cord

Compressive lower cervical or upper thoracic myelopathy may produce spastic paraplegia with a mid-thoracic sensory level (or "girdle sensation").[27,28] For example, in one case a spastic paraplegia with a sensory level at T10 was associated with cervical compression from a herniated disc at C5/C6.[29]

Radiculopathy

False localising radiculopathy may occur in the context of IIH and cerebral venous sinus thrombosis, manifesting as acral paraesthesias, backache and radicular pain, and less often with motor deficits,[30] which on occasion may be sufficiently extensive to mimic Guillain-Barré syndrome (flaccid-areflexic quadriplegia).[31] The postulated mechanism for such radiculopathy is mechanical root compression due to elevated CSF pressure. However, acute radiculopathies have also been described in cases of intracranial hypotension.[32,33]

Higher cortical functions

Dysarthria in the absence of aphasia ("pure dysarthria") may occur on occasion with cortical infarction in the anterior internal capsule or corona radiata, sometimes with an isolated facial paresis.[34] This is presumably cognate with the syndrome described as "cortical dysarthria" which could also be associated with transient facial weakness.[35]

Hemineglect is much commoner with right rather than left parietal lobe lesions. An example of false-localising neglect has been encountered: in a patient with a posterior fossa meningioma causing left pontine compression, long tract signs and hydrocephalus, ipsilesional neglect was found, despite normal structural imaging of the cerebral hemispheres. The neglect resolved promptly after shunting and did not recur despite progressive brainstem compression (PC Nachev & IH Jenkins, personal communication).

Comment

As false-localising signs most often occur in the context of RICP, this seems likely to be the most important factor in the pathogenesis of these signs. Suggested mechanisms include mechanical distortion of cranial nerves with intracranial pathology and venous and/or arterial ischaemia with spinal cord pathology.[3] It is worth remembering that RICP itself may be a false localising sign when associated with spinal tumours, even in the thoracolumbar region, perhaps related to elevated CSF protein concentration.[36]

Of the various false-localising signs described, sixth nerve palsies are the most commonly observed. Some argue that abducens nerve palsy is the only acceptable false localising sign in IIH,[37] and certainly investigation for other causes of cranial nerve palsy is mandatory in these situations. However, the possibility of false localisation should be borne in mind when any of the above-mentioned signs occur without obvious clinical-anatomical or clinical-radiological correlate.[2] But such false localisation is rare, indeed exceptional, and does not invalidate teaching rules regarding the localisation of neurological lesions generally.

Acknowledgement

Adapted and updated from: Larner AJ. False localising signs. *J Neurol Neurosurg Psychiatry* 2003;74:415–418; Larner AJ. A topographical anatomy of false-localising signs. *Adv Clin Neurosci Rehabil* 2005;5(1):20–21.

References

1. Collier J. *The false localising signs of intracranial tumour.* Brain 1904;27:490–508.
2. Larner AJ. *A dictionary of neurological signs* (4th edition). London: Springer, 2016.
3. Larner AJ. *False localising signs.* J Neurol Neurosurg Psychiatry 2003;74:415–418.
4. Kernohan JW, Woltman HW. *Incisura of the crus due to contralateral brain tumor.* Arch Neurol Psychiatry 1929;21:274–287.
5. Cohen AR, Wilson J. *Magnetic resonance imaging of Kernohan's notch.* Neurosurgery 1990;27:205–207.
6. Zhang CH, DeSouza RM, Kho JSB, Vundavalli S, Critchley G. *Kernohan-Woltman notch phenomenon: a review article.* Br J Neurosurg 2017;31:159–166.
7. Gado M, Hanaway J, Frank R. *Functional anatomy of the cerebral cortex by computed tomography.* J Comput Assist Tomog 1979;3:1–19.
8. Schulz R, Fegbeutel C, Althoff A, Traupe H, Grimminger F, Seeger W. *Central

sleep apnoea and unilateral diaphragmatic paralysis associated with vertebral artery compression of the medulla oblongata. J Neurol 2003;250:503–505.

9. Hiraga A, Kojima K, Suzuki M, Kuwabara S. *Isolated contralateral spinothalamic sensory loss below thoracic level due to lateral medullary infarction.* Acta Neurol Belg 2024;124:279–281.

10. Marshman LAG, Polkey CE, Penney CC. *Unilateral fixed dilation of the pupil as a false-localizing sign with intracranial hemorrhage: case report and literature review.* Neurosurgery 2001;49:1251–1255.

11. Ksiazek SM, Repka MX, Maguire A et al. *Divisional oculomotor nerve paresis caused by intrinsic brainstem disease.* Ann Neurol 1989;26:714–718.

12. Larner AJ. *Proximal superior division oculomotor nerve palsy from metastatic subarachnoid infiltration.* J Neurol 2002;249:343–344.

13. Rezazadeh A, Rohani M. *Idiopathic intracranial hypertension with complete oculomotor palsy.* Neurol India 2010;58:820–821.

14. Lee AG. *Fourth nerve palsy in pseudotumor cerebri.* Strabismus 1995;3:57–59.

15. Speer C, Pearlman J, Phillips PH et al. *Fourth nerve palsy in pediatric pseudotumor cerebri.* Am J Ophthalmol 1999;127:236–237.

16. Arsava EM, Uluc K, Nurlu G, Kansu T. *Electrophysiological evidence of trigeminal neuropathy in pseudotumor cerebri.* J Neurol 2002;249:1601–1602.

17. Matsuura N, Kondo A. *Trigeminal neuralgia and hemifacial spasm as false localizing signs in patients with a contralateral mass of the posterior cranial fossa.* J Neurosurg 1996;84:1067–1071.

18. Kandoh T, Tamaki N, Takeda N, Shirataki K, Matsumoto S. *Contralateral trigeminal neuralgia as a false localizing sign in calcified chronic subdural hematoma: a case report.* Surg Neurol 1989;32:471–475.

19. Round R, Keane JR. *The minor symptoms of increased intracranial pressure. 101 cases with benign intracranial hypertension.* Neurology 1988;38:1461–1464.

20. Davie C, Kennedy P, Katifi HA. *Seventh nerve palsy as a false localising sign.* J Neurol Neurosurg Psychiatry 1992;55:510–511.

21. Kiwak KJ, Levine SE. *Benign intracranial hypertension and facial diplegia.* Arch Neurol 1984;41:787–788.

22. Dorman PJ, Campbell MJ, Maw AR. *Hearing loss as a false localising sign in raised intracranial pressure.* J Neurol Neurosurg Psychiatry 1995;58:516.

23. Ro LS, Chen ST, Tang LM et al. *Concurrent trigeminal, abducens, and facial nerve palsies presenting as false localizing signs.* Neurosurgery 1995;37:322–324.

24. Maurice-Williams RS. *Multiple crossed false localizing signs in a posterior fossa tumour.* J Neurol Neurosurg Psychiatry 1975;38:1232–1234.

25. Willoughby E, Anderson N. *Lower cranial nerve motor function in unilateral vascular lesions of the cerebral hemisphere.* BMJ 1984;289:791–794.

26. Sonstein WJ, LaSala PA, Michelsen WJ et al. *False localizing signs in upper cervical spinal cord compression.* Neurosurgery 1996;38:445–448.

27. Adams KK, Jackson CE, Rauch RA, Hart SF, Kleinguenther RS, Barohn RJ.

Cervical myelopathy with false localizing sensory levels. Arch Neurol 1996;53:1155–1158.

28. Ochiai H, Yamakawa Y, Minato S, Nakahara K, Nakano S, Wakisaka S. *Clinical features of the localized girdle sensation of mid-trunk (false localizing sign) appeared [sic] in cervical compressive myelopathy patients.* J Neurol 2002;249:549–553.

29. Pego-Regiosa R, Trobajo de las Matas JE, Brañas F, Martinez-Vázquez F, Cortés-Laíño JA. *Dorsal sensory level as a false localizing sign in cervical myelopathy* [in Spanish]. Rev Neurol 1998;27:86–88.

30. Moosa A, Joy MA, Kumar A. *Extensive radiculopathy: another false localising sign in intracranial hypertension.* J Neurol Neurosurg Psychiatry 2004;75:1080–1081.

31. Obeid T, Awada A, Mousali Y et al. *Extensive radiculopathy: a manifestation of intracranial hypertension.* Eur J Neurol 2000;7:549–553.

32. Albayram S, Wasserman BA, Yousem DM, Wityk R. *Intracranial hypotension as a cause of radiculopathy from epidural cervical venous engorgement: a case report.* AJNR 2002;23:618–621.

33. Kleopa KA, Natsiopoulos K. *Acute cervical radiculopathies in spontaneous intracranial hypotension.* J Neurol 2009;256:499–501.

34. Tanaka K, Yamada T, Torii T et al. *Pure dysarthria and dysarthria-facial paresis syndrome due to internal capsule and/or corona radiata infarction.* BMC Neurol 2015;15:184.

35. Whitty CWM. *Cortical dysarthria and prosody of speech.* J Neurol Neurosurg Psychiatry 1964;27:507–510.

36. Ridsdale L, Moseley I. *Thoracolumbar intraspinal tumour presenting features of raised intracranial pressure.* J Neurol Neurosurg Psychiatry 1978;41:737–745.

37. Menon RN, Radhakrishnan K. *Idiopathic intracranial hypertension: are false localising signs other than abducens nerve palsy acceptable?* Neurol India 2010;58:683–684.

"Flamingo test"

As all ornithologists know, the six species of flamingo (Phoenicopteriformes or Phoenicopteridae) are far from the only birds to roost standing on one leg, but nevertheless it is these birds alone who seem to have been co-opted by clinicians to describe the single leg stance (e.g. in radiology[1]). Whereas birds can sustain this posture for hours, and whilst asleep, its adoption is more challenging for humans.

The 10–second one leg standing (10s-OLS) test, colloquially known as the "flamingo test," has been demonstrated to have utility for mortality risk assessment by Araujo et al.[2] Failure to achieve 10s-OLS ("NO 10s-OLS") was found to be associated with patient age, high waist-height ratio, and prevalence of diabetes mellitus.[2] The 10s-OLS test is attractive for clinical use since it is easily administered, safe, and simply categorised (binary yes/no), so should be easy to apply in practice.

Contrary to the view expressed by Araujo et al. that "balance assessment is not routinely incorporated in the clinical examination",[2] most neurologists would include such an assessment in their neurological examination, particularly in older patients,[3] and invariably if there is a complaint of imbalance or falling. Hence for neurologists, the findings of the study of the "flamingo test" beg questions about underlying neurobiological mechanisms. Aside from speculating that "subclinical central or autonomic nervous system dysfunction" might contribute, the authors do not specifically address these issues, other than to indicate the exclusion from their study of patients with unstable gait or with signs of acute vestibular or otoneurological disturbance.[2]

Age-related changes in balance-control are common, involving both sensory systems (somatosensory [proprioceptive], visual, and vestibular inputs) and motor systems (strength, range of motion, coordination), as well as cognitive functions (sensory adaptation, attention).[3] Any or all of these factors might contribute to the clinical finding of NO 10s-OLS. Whilst associated with factors which might suggest that cerebrovascular disease is a significant contributor, such as high waist-height ratio and prevalence of diabetes mellitus, and hence potentially amenable to intervention, this will not be the case for all patients.

Fractionation of NO 10s-OLS patients by means of screening and/or formal neurological examination will surely be necessary if the findings of Araujo et al. are to lead to meaningful, individualised, interventions to reduce mortality. This examination might include the modified Romberg test to assess proprioceptive, visual, and vestibular inputs,[4] as well as assessment of motor strength and coordination.

Acknowledgement

Adapted from: Larner AJ. Re: Successful 10–second one-legged stance predicts survival in middle-aged and older individuals.
https://bjsm.bmj.com/content/early/2022/06/22/bjsports-2021–105360.responses (Published 26 June 2022)

References

1. Garras DN, Carothers JT, Olson SA. Single-leg-stance (flamingo) radiographs to assess pelvic instability: how much motion is normal? J Bone Joint Surg Am 2008; 90: 2114–8.
2. Araujo CG, de Souza e Silva CG, Laukkanen JA et al. Successful 10–second one-legged stance predicts survival in middle-aged and older individuals. Br J Sports Med 2022; 56: 975–80.
3. Schott JM, Larner AJ. Neurological signs of ageing. In: Sinclair AJ, Morley JE, Villas B, Cesare M, Munshi M (eds). *Pathy's Principles and Practice of Geriatric Medicine.* 6th edition. Wiley Blackwell, 2022: 563–569. https://doi.org/10.1002/9781119484288.ch44
4. Agrawal Y, Carey JP, Hoffman HJ, Sklare DA, Schubert MC. The modified Romberg balance test: normative data in US adults. Otol Neurotol 2011; 32: 1309–11.

Glossorrhoea or logorrhoea?

"I never heard or read of any body with such a severely copious chronic glossorhoea [*sic*]."[1]

Thus, Thomas Henry Huxley (1825–95) opining on William Gladstone, then in his first stint as Prime Minister, in September 1871.

All clinicians are familiar with the prefix "glosso-" denoting tongue, as in glossodynia (pain in the tongue, as in burning mouth syndrome), glossolalia (speaking in tongues),[2] and glossophobia (fear of public speaking). Likewise the suffix "-rrhoea" denoting a superfluity or excess flow of, as in diarrhoea (of faeces), rhinorrhoea or otorrhoea (of CSF from nose or ear, respectively), sialorrhoea (saliva), seborrhoea (of sebum, as in Parkinson's disease); and there are other examples (dysmenorrhoea, galactorrhoea, gonorrhoea). So why not glossorrhoea?

Whether or not the (clinically unqualified) Huxley was coining a neologism, his meaning seems unequivocal: a superfluity of tongue, implying Gladstone says too much (rich, coming from a man who was, quite evidently from his biography, never short of something to say or write). This, then, was not used by Huxley to define a clinical entity, but as a term of ridicule or abuse.

Perhaps understandably, then, I do not recall use of "glossorrhoea" during my years of clinical practice, but from time to time have encountered a related term: logorrhoea. Again, the prefix, "logo-", is familiar, as in logopenia (for example the logopenic aphasic variant of Alzheimer disease) and logoclonia (reiterating the final syllable of words).[3]

Logorrhoea is thus extreme loquacity, or "incessant incoherent talking" as one nineteenth-century clinician, Robert Lawson, described "Mania associated with logorrhoea", such that "Any substance capable of putting a stop to the logorrhoea prevalent in both the male and female wards of an asylum would be of immense advantage in asylum management".[4] This definition may therefore overlap with glossorrhoea; or an excessive verbal output, implying pressure of speech, as in certain psychiatric conditions. If the verbal output is in any way incoherent, then this may imply an aphasic syndrome, particularly a Wernicke type aphasia in which neologisms may be evident, sometimes denoted by terminology such word salad, verbigeration, or jargon (a term used by Hughlings Jackson[5]).

To my knowledge, little has been published on logorrhoea as a clinical entity per se,[6] as opposed to its use as a pejorative term,[7,8] as for Huxley's use of glossorrhoea. The one study of which I am aware reported on verbal production by normal subjects reading speeches, finding that degree of education exerted an effect whereas age and sex did not (might this have been different if spontaneous speech had been analysed?). In patients with frontotemporal lobar degeneration and logorrhoea, structural neuroimaging suggested atrophy was most frequently observed in anteroinferior and anteromedial regions of the right temporal lobe.[6]

Acknowledgement

Unpublished manuscript, mid-2023.

References

1. Desmond A. *Huxley: from devil's disciple to evolution's high priest.* London: Penguin, 1998: 423.
2. Larner AJ. *A dictionary of neurological signs* (4th edition). London: Springer; 2016: 141–142.
3. Op. cit., ref. 2: 190.
4. Lawson R. Hyoscyamine in the treatment of some diseases of the insane. *West Riding Lunatic Asylum Medical Reports* 1876; 6: 65–84 [at 67, 77].
5. Jackson JH. On affections of speech from disease of the brain. *Brain* 1879–1880; 2: 323–356.
6. Robles-Bayón A, Santos-Garcia D, Rodríguez-Osorio X, Sánchez-Salom A, Barandela-Salgado J, Fernández-Ferro JC. A clinico-anatomical correlation study of logorrhoea [in Spanish]. *Rev Neurol* 2009; 49: 633–638.
7. Persson PB. One hundred thousand US dollars to battle scientific logorrhoea. *Acta Physiol (Oxf)* 2018 Mar; 222(3). doi:10.1111/apha.12991.
8. Looi JC, Anderson K. COVID-19 isolated-academic logorrhoea: an emergent debilitating disorder afflicting medical academics. *Australas Psychiatry* 2021; 29: 104–105.

Intracranial bruit

When performing a neurological examination, should you auscultate for intracranial bruits over the skull, and/or the orbits? The notional purpose of such an examination is to identify an underlying arteriovenous malformation or dural arteriovenous fistula, turbulent blood flow in the shunt producing a bruit detectable with the stethoscope. But there is little, if any, evidence to recommend this procedure. The founding editor of the journal *Practical Neurology*, Charles Warlow, writing with a number of his colleagues in the second edition of their textbook of stroke medicine, published 20 years ago, opined that:

> The general examination provides rather few clues to the cause of an intracerebral haemorrhage ... Auscultating the skull for detecting arterio-venous malformations is useful for impressing naïve readers of textbooks as well as medical students and patients, but is not very rewarding.[1]

In light of this, the following challenge was issued, in the form of an offer:

> We are still waiting for someone, who had no other clues and only by auscultation diagnosed an arteriovenous malformation in an adult, to take up our offer of a free copy of this book.[1]

I have no information as to whether or not this challenge was ever successfully answered and the prize claimed, but I would suspect not. Likewise, I would anticipate that most readers would answer my introductory question in the negative.

Certainly I was surprised when, after publishing with colleagues a case report describing rapid cognitive decline in a patient subsequently diagnosed with a dural arteriovenous fistula,[2] a rare but recognised cause of reversible cognitive impairment,[3] I received communication from the journal editor inviting a response to a correspondent who asked whether or not we had performed skull auscultation.[4]

How might one make a meaningful reply to this enquiry, other than "No, we did not", when there are no empirical data, not even a single diagnostic test accuracy study, let alone multiple studies suitable for systematic review and meta-analysis?

A possible approach is one couched in terms of binary classification, that is, examining the implications of the 2x2 contingency table for a diagnostic test accuracy study.[5] This assumes that a methodologically robust test accuracy study of skull auscultation could be undertaken. The index test could perhaps be standardised to listening in specified cranial locations and for specified durations, and the reference ("gold") standard for diagnosis of arteriovenous malformation or fistula might be a specified modality of brain imaging. Hence a 2x2 contingency table could be constructed.

Making the assumption, hopefully not unreasonable, that intracranial bruits constitute a rare clinical sign, a policy of routinely auscultating the skull in all patients would occasion many true negatives, particularly if there were "no other clues". The same would probably also be true even in the presence of clinical pointers, which might perhaps include suspected intracranial haemorrhage or subacute cognitive decline. Likewise, very few false positives (i.e. hearing a bruit in the absence of an arteriovenous malformation or fistula) would be anticipated. Hence, with many true negatives and very few false positives one would anticipate very high test specificity for intracranial bruit. Following the "SpPin" heuristic[6] – that for a highly Specific test, a Positive test rules the diagnosis in – any bruit would likely be diagnostic.

Considering test sensitivity, any assumptions would be a little more tentative. Nevertheless one might suspect that in patients with proven arteriovenous malformation or fistula false negatives (no bruit heard) would be more common than true positives if the skull is not a good transmitter (i.e. an effective filter) of the sound of a bruit. If this assumption were correct, the result would be low test sensitivity. With very few true positives and even fewer false positives, positive predictive value might be quite high, but with wide confidence intervals.

Since true negatives also feature in the numerator of both negative predictive value and correct classification accuracy, one might anticipate that, because of the overwhelming preponderance of true negatives, these parameters would be inflated. Indeed this is a situation in which a more meaningful metric to assess the value of a diagnostic test might be one which ignores true negatives, such as the critical success index (or threat score) or the F measure,[7] the latter widely used in information retrieval and machine learning contexts but less familiar in the clinical literature.

Another option might be to construct a receiver operating characteristic (ROC) curve, which plots sensitivity (true positive rate) against false positive rate (= 1 − Specificity), with the area under the curve used as the measure of diagnostic accuracy. However, because the sign under investigation is a binary classifier, the "curve" would in fact be a single point, a ROC dot rather than plot, with the test accuracy measure given by the area under a triangle rather than area under a curve.[8]

As chance would have it, since writing my response to the journal, I have come across an account which might be viewed as the exception which proves the rule (or, more correctly, the regularity), and hence the wisdom of Warlow's challenge. It emanates from no less an authority than a Nobel Prize winner (in Medicine/Physiology in 1981), David H. Hubel (1926–2013), who qualified in medicine before pursuing his career in visual neurophysiology, mostly in collaboration with Torsten N. Wiesel. Recalling his days as a junior doctor on the neurology service at Johns Hopkins Hospital in Baltimore, circa 1954, Hubel reports:

> The chief of neurology, Jack Magladery, cultivated an eccentric bedside manner. He always began his neurological examination of a patient by listening to the eye with a stethoscope, never hearing anything but always impressing onlookers. One night I was prowling around the medical wards looking for interesting cases when one of the medical interns brought me to see a patient who was a major puzzle, with a hemiparesis and an assortment of other symptoms that I can't remember, and in any case made no sense to anyone. I began examining him, and because a few house staff were looking on I started by listening to the eyes. To my amazement, from one of the eyes came a noise like a pulsating fire hose, a bruit the likes of which I had never heard before, and which made it immediately clear that this man's problem was a cerebral arteriovenous shunt. So suddenly there were crowds of interns and residents around the bed, and I had been catapulted to instant fame. That cancelled out any number of previous blunders.[9]

Interestingly, Magladery did publish on cerebrovascular haemorrhage, but made no mention of auscultation or intracranial bruits.[10]

Whether Hubel's example would (prospectively!) meet Warlow's challenge is moot. Would the hemiparesis count as a clue? Certainly it appears from the (retrospective) account that diagnosis was "only by auscultation". Nevertheless, this clinical anecdote provides no evidence against, and indeed further evidence in favour of, Charles Warlow's view that "Auscultating the skull for detecting arteriovenous malformations is useful for impressing naïve readers of textbooks as well as medical students and patients, but is not very rewarding".[1]

Acknowledgement

Adapted from: Larner AJ. Intracranial bruit: Charles Warlow's challenge revisited. *Pract Neurol* 2022;22:79–81.

References

1. Warlow C, Dennis M, van Gijn J et al. *Stroke A practical guide to management* (2nd edition). Oxford: Blackwell Publishing; 2001;360.
2. Randall A, Ellis R, Hywel B, Davies RR, Alusi SH, Larner AJ. Rapid cognitive decline: not always Creutzfeldt-Jakob disease. *J R Coll Physicians Edinb* 2015;45:209–12.
3. Wilson M, Doran M, Enevoldsen TP, Larner AJ. Cognitive profiles associated with intracranial dural arteriovenous fistula. *Age Ageing* 2010;39:389–92.
4. Lowenthal MN. Auscultation of the skull. *J R Coll Physicians Edinb* 2016;46:214.
5. Larner AJ. Auscultation of the skull: author's reply. *J R Coll Physicians Edinb* 2016;46:214.
6. Strauss SE, Glasziou P, Richardson WS, Haynes RB. *Evidence-based medicine. How to practice and teach EBM* (5th edition). Edinburgh: Elsevier; 2019;165–6.
7. Larner AJ. Assessing cognitive screeners with the critical success index. *Prog Neurol Psychiatry* 2021;25(3):33–7.
8. Mbizvo GK, Larner AJ. Receiver operating characteristic plot and area under the curve with binary classifiers: pragmatic analysis of cognitive screening instruments. *Neurodegener Dis Manag* 2021;11:353–60.
9. Hubel DH, Wiesel TN. *Brain and visual perception. The story of a 25–year collaboration.* Oxford: Oxford University Press; 2005;16.
10. Magladery JW. The natural course of cerebrovascular hemorrhage. *Clin Neurosurg* 1963;9:106–13.

Jaw Jerk

The jaw jerk, or masseter reflex, is contraction of the masseter and temporalis muscles in response to a light tap on the chin with a tendon hammer with the mouth held slightly open and with the mandibular muscles relaxed. Both the afferent and efferent limbs of the reflex arc run in the mandibular division of the trigeminal (V) nerve, connecting centrally with the mesencephalic (motor) nucleus of the trigeminal nerve. The reflex is highly reproducible; there is a linear correlation between age and reflex latency, and a negative correlation between age and reflex amplitude. Interruption of the reflex arc leads to a diminished or absent jaw jerk as in bulbar palsy (although an absent jaw jerk may be a normal finding, particularly in older persons). Bilateral supranuclear lesions cause a brisk jaw jerk, as in pseudobulbar palsy (*e.g.* in motor neurone disease).[1]

The original description of the jaw jerk reflex has sometimes been attributed to Armand de Watteville (1846–1925), a physician perhaps best known for his editorship of *Brain: a journal of neurology* (1884–1901) and his key role in inaugurating the Neurological Society of London (1885–6).[2] Through his interest in electrotherapeutics (he held an appointment in this department at St. Mary's Hospital, London) he had also taken an interest in the physiology of the knee jerk reflex, a new addition to the neurological examination as of 1875 and a subject of interest and research for many clinicians.[3,4] Using an apparatus designed by Augustus Desiré Waller (1856–1922), de Watteville was able to record both tendon percussion and muscle contraction, but initially arrived at no definite conclusion as to the exact nature of the knee jerk.[5] Later he concluded, erroneously that these were "tendon reactions" or "myotatic contractions", hence a "pseudo-reflex", a local mechanical response consequent on sudden muscle stretching, rather than a true reflex.[6]

de Watteville's claim for priority with respect to the jaw jerk is based on a note published in the January 1886 issue of *Brain*.[7] In this note he called "the attention of neurologists" to the fact that a "jaw-jerk" could be readily elicited by an appropriate stimulus in most healthy persons. "The phenomenon is clearly of the same nature as that of the 'knee-jerk', and is due to the sudden stretching of the masseter and other muscles of mastication. Hence the name I have ventured to give to it [jaw-jerk], in preference to the longer and less accurate term mandibular (or masseteric) tendon-reaction (or reflex)". His clinical observation was that "In many cases, especially in such where one finds the usual tendon-reactions exaggerated, one readily obtains a very lively jaw-jerk". Moreover, "This fact, I feel bound to state, was quite familiar to me before it came to my knowledge that the phenomenon had been observed in a case in America. I have not been able to ascertain the author of, any details about, nor the reference to, this observation". His electrophysiological investigations attempting to record the jaw jerk suggested to de Watteville that its latency was too short to be compatible with a reflex, and hence as for the knee-jerk he considered it to be a consequence of direct stimulation of the muscles.

de Watteville's note was in fact a response to a paper by Charles Beevor (1854–1908) describing jaw clonus in a case of motor neurone disease.[8] Beevor reported that he had been alerted by William Gowers (1845–1915) to "a case published in America, in which an increased tendon-reflex of the muscles of the lower jaw was obtained". Beevor's patient had bulbar paralysis and the "knee-jerks were excessive on both sides".

As regards the "case published in America", de Watteville noted that "Both Dr. Gower's [sic] and Dr. Beevor's information concerning this case is limited to the bare fact of its existence". Knowing of Gowers' antipathy to de Watteville (Gowers did not publish in *Brain* for the duration of de Watteville's editorship, nor did he join the Neurological Society of London, apparently considering de Watteville a charlatan[9]), we can be certain that there was no direct communication between the two to clarify this point.

As shown by Lanska,[10] Fine and Lohr,[11,12] and Pearce,[13] the "case published in America" referred to a report by Morris James Lewis (1852–1928) which appeared in the 9th May 1885 issue of *The Medical and Surgical Reporter*, a journal published in Philadelphia.[14] Lewis observed what he termed the "chin reflex", initially in November 1882, in a "case of section of the inferior dental nerve" seen at the Infirmary for Nervous Diseases in Philadelphia. Since then, he had "observed this symptom in two cases of spastic paralysis, one case of congestion of the spinal cord, one of cerebral tumor, probably specific, one of hemiplegia, one of unilateral tumour of doubtful origin, and occasionally in perfectly healthy individuals" (cf. differences from the quotations presented in Fine & Lohr's abstract[11]).

Lewis later published with Silas Weir Mitchell on the knee jerk.[3] As Physician to the Infirmary for Nervous Diseases and to the Children's Hospital, he also published a note on the use of eucalyptus in headache.[15]

Acknowledgement

Unpublished manuscript, November-December 2024.

References

1. Larner AJ. *A dictionary of neurological signs* (4th edition). London: Springer, 2016: 178.
2. Larner AJ, Triarhou LC. Armand de Watteville (1846–1925). *J Neurol* 2025; 272: 136.
3. Lazar JW. The early history of the knee-jerk reflex in neurology. *J Hist Neurosci* 2022; 31: 409–424.
4. Adan G, Larner AJ. Sesquicentenary of the knee jerk reflex: the contributions of Hughlings Jackson, Horsley, and Sherrington. *J Hist Neurosci* (in press).
5. de Watteville A. On reflexes and pseudo-reflexes. *BMJ* 1882; 1: 736–737.
6. de Watteville A. On the tendon-reactions. *BMJ* 1886; 1: 1160.
7. de Watteville A. Note on the jaw-jerk, or masseteric tendon reaction, in health and disease. *Brain* 1885–1886; 8: 518–519.
8. Beevor CE. A case of amyotrophic lateral sclerosis with clonus of the lower jaw. *Brain* 1885–1886; 8: 516–518.
9. Hunting P. *The history of the Royal Society of Medicine*. London: Royal Society of Medicine Press, 2002.
10. Lanska DJ. Morris James Lewis (1852–1928) and the description of the jaw jerk. *J Child Neurol* 1991; 6: 235–236.
11. Fine EJ, Lohr L. Morris J. Lewis discovered the jaw jerk reflex in 1885. Presentation to the Fifth Annual Meeting of the International Society for the History of the Neurosciences, Providence, Rhode Island, USA, 13 June 2000.
12. Fine EJ, Lohr LA. The chin reflex. *Muscle Nerve* 2003; 27: 386.
13. Pearce JM. The jaw jerk: an instance of misattribution. *J Neurol Neurosurg Psychiatry* 2011; 82: 351–352.
14. Lewis MJ. The chin reflex. A new clinical observation. *Med Surg Reporter* 1885; 52 (19). 591 (9th May).
15. Lewis MJ, De Schweinitz GE. A preliminary note on the use of eucalyptus in headache. *The Medical News* 1889; 55(3): 62–63 (20th July).

"Migramnesia"

Introduction

Transient global amnesia (TGA), a self-limiting episode of dense anterograde amnesia often characterised by repetitive circular questioning and with a variable duration of retrograde amnesia, was first described as such in the 1950s.[1] The exact pathophysiology of TGA remains undefined.[2] However, an association between migraine diathesis and the predisposition to TGA is long-established and robustly confirmed, extending from initial individual case reports and case series to more recent population-based studies.[3,4] In addition to acting as a predisposing factor for TGA, typical amnesic episodes have sometimes been described in the context of an episode of migraine headache, suggesting that migraine might also on occasion act as a precipitating or triggering factor for TGA. The frequency and symptomatology of this concurrence is ill-defined, in part because classification schemata such as the International Classification of Headache Disorders 3rd edition (ICHD3) do not recognise amnesia or memory loss symptoms in association with migraine,[5] and TGA criteria accept headache as a common "non-focal" incidental feature in TGA episodes.[6]

In order to reappraise the clinical phenomena of migraine and TGA occurring in close temporal association, three illustrative cases are presented in light of which the aims of the discussion are to review the previous literature on migraine as a precipitating factor for TGA, and for other paroxysmal events such as epilepsy and stroke; to consider possible shared pathophysiological mechanisms which might explain why in these circumstances subsequence is indeed consequence; and hence to suggest the term "migramnesia" as an appropriate way to denote this clinical scenario.

Case 1

A 75 year-old lady was referred to the neurology clinic following an episode in which she lost her memory for about an hour. The history from the patient and her daughter was that they were together at her home one morning. She chatted on the phone with a relative, mentioning her anxiety about an upcoming hospital appointment. She also complained of some head pain for which she took paracetamol. Thereafter she was forgetful, could not recall things that had happened in the previous week, and subsequently had no recall of her conversations either with her daughter or the telephone call made during this time period. When seen in the neurology clinic about 3 months later, this event was judged to conform to the clinical diagnostic criteria for TGA,[6] as there was evidence of both anterograde and retrograde amnesia.

About fourteen years earlier, aged 62, the patient had had an episode of amnesia lasting several hours; this occurred on Boxing Day and she was unable to recall events of the previous Christmas Day. Brain imaging (MR) and EEG performed about one month after this episode showed no abnormalities. The neurologist who assessed the patient at this time had made a diagnosis of TGA.

Her past medical history also included a thirty-year history of episodic throbbing headaches above the right eye, symptoms ascribed by the patient to 'sinus trouble' but judged retrospectively to be typical of migraine.

Case 2

A 57 year-old lady who suffered about 3 episodes of migraine each year, usually responsive to paracetamol, was referred for assessment of an amnesic episode following a typical migraine. The day after returning from an overseas holiday, the flight arriving in the early hours of the morning, she developed a headache for which she took paracetamol and went to bed. About 3 hours later, she woke and was asking family members repetitive questions about what was going on; she had no recall of the flight, and could not remember her current car, naming one that she had owned thirty years previously. The memory symptoms improved after about 3 hours but she was left with an amnesic gap of about 24 hours, although she could recall details of the holiday. Brain imaging (MR) performed about six months after the amnesic episode showed no abnormalities. Subsequent neurological opinion judged the episode to conform to the clinical diagnostic criteria for TGA.[6]

Case 3

A 65 year-old lady who had suffered from episodic migraine with aura since young adulthood was referred following an episode of memory loss occurring in the context of prolonged constant headache. This was more severe than her usual episodic migraines and was associated with phonophobia and occasional episodes of her typical visual aura. About four weeks after headache onset, for most of one day she had no clear recollection of her activities, including getting up, washing and dressing, driving, or attending a job interview. Collateral history from the interview noted she gave short responses to questions, a behaviour recognised to be out of character. She was able to drive home thereafter, where her daughter observed repetitive questioning but no other symptoms. By the time the patient attended the local A&E department in the evening, the memory symptoms were improving. Although she could recall no headache that day, the medical staff treated her with a triptan. Brain imaging (CT) was normal. Interval MR brain imaging, about 3 weeks later, was also unremarkable. Subsequent neurological opinion judged the amnesic episode to conform to the clinical criteria for TGA.[6]

Discussion

These three patients experienced criterial episodes of TGA occurring in the temporal context of migraine headache without visual or somatosensory aura.

Transient impairment or loss of memory has long been recognised as an attendant feature in some migraine attacks: they were mentioned, for example, in Liveing's monograph of 1873 which also referred to earlier cases described by Tissot and by Parry.[7] Moersch in 1924 emphasized amnestic dysfunction occurring in migraine attacks,[8] and Nielsen in 1958 wrote of the "amnesia of migraine" although none of the five cases he described (nos. 29–33) had a clinical phenotype now recognisable as that of TGA.[9] Frank in 1976 compared amnesic episodes in migraine, which he termed "Migranedammerattacken", with reports of TGA and suggested that they seemed to be identical.[10] A syndrome of acute confusional migraine in children has been noted to have clinical features similar to TGA,[11] prompting the idea of "cognitive migraine".[12]

Whilst the association between migraine and TGA is robustly established for a history of migraine tendency, hence as a predisposing factor,[13] TGA occurring in the context of a migraine episode, hence migraine as a precipitating or triggering factor, is less frequently noted. There are occasional case reports and series describing patients in whom an episode of migraine was followed by TGA,[14,15] some in apparently familial cases of TGA.[16,17] Cases are also described wherein TGA is followed immediately by a typical migraine headache such that TGA is considered to be migraine aura,[18,19] some with the typical MR imaging signature of hippocampal CA1 area punctate hyperintensities seen in many TGA cases.[20] However, both of these categories are relatively infrequently reported, so might possibly be ascribed to nothing more than chance concurrence. The only study in a defined population, a retrospective analysis of a cohort of 8821 new patients seen over an 11–year period in a dedicated migraine clinical centre in France, reported only 6 cases of TGA "triggered" by a migraine attack.[21] These data prompted the view, in a recent monograph devoted to TGA, that "TGA occurring during a migraine attack ... is probably a very rare occurrence".[22]

However, a number of confounding factors may be operating here which might negate, or modify, this conclusion. There may be under-reporting, and possibly underascertainment, of TGA: as a transient self-limiting condition, patients may not present to neurological attention (or only very late, as in our cases) and/or the absence of reliable collateral history may render the clinical diagnosis unavailable since the clinical diagnostic criteria are by application binary ("definite or pure TGA" or "not TGA"). But even if TGA is reported and ascertained, there may be under-reporting and possibly underascertainment of migraine occurring as a feature of TGA. This may be simply a consequence of accepting headache as an incidental feature in TGA episodes, which reportedly occurs in around 10% of cases.[6,23,24]

In addition to these considerations, one also needs to consider the nature of TGA itself. If a *sine qua non* of TGA is a period of retrograde amnesia (although not criterial[6]), then patients will by definition not recall events such as migraine aura and/or headache occurring immediately before the onset of anterograde amnesia (see, for example, our Case 3), as these events may fall within the resulting amnesic gap. Hence one is dependent on the collateral history from a reliable informant, which may understandably focus on the memory symptoms, as more dramatic, unfamiliar, and hence concerning (e.g. of a stroke) rather than headache symptoms, particularly if the patient is already known to have a tendency to migraine. Thus, if not specifically enquired for, migraine as a precipitating or triggering factor for TGA may be easily overlooked.

Migraine as a trigger for other neurological phenomena is well recognised, albeit relatively uncommon. For example, in 1960 the American epileptologist William G. Lennox (1884–1960) coined the term "migralepsy" to describe a clinical scenario in which "ophthalmic migraine with perhaps nausea and vomiting was followed by symptoms characteristic of epilepsy".[25] The concept of migralepsy has proved controversial, with some authorities advocating abolition of the term in favour of "ictal epileptic headache",[26] although migralepsy is enshrined in ICHD3 as a "seizure triggered by an attack of migraine with aura" with specific diagnostic criteria.[5] It is also recognised that migraine features may sometimes be followed by stroke. Denoted as migraine stroke or, as per ICHD3 terminology, migrainous infarction, this is defined as "one or more migraine aura symptoms occurring in association with an ischaemic brain lesion in the appropriate territory demonstrated by neuroimaging, with onset during the course of a typical migraine with aura attack".[5]

Could a mechanistic explanation of migraine followed by TGA, or of TGA as a form of migraine aura, be posited? Just as shared mechanisms have been postulated to explain the differing clinical features in migralepsy[27] and in migrainous infarction,[28] the same may be the case for migraine and TGA. Specifically, the mechanism of cortical spreading depression, also known as spreading depolarization, has long been suggested as the cause of both migraine aura and TGA,[29] and this remains a favoured explanation for the observed clinical phenomena of TGA.[2,30] Spread of depolarization from occipital to temporal cortex might explain the sequential clinical phenomena of migraine and amnesia, or from temporal to occipital cortex to explain TGA as a migraine aura.

In light of such considerations we suggest, following Lennox's characterisation of "migralepsy",[25] that the term "migramnesia" be used to denote this particular concatenation of neurological events. Rather than coining a needless neologism, a key advantage of this proposed nomenclature is that it characterises headache as potentially integral, rather than merely incidental, to episodes of TGA. If this term is used in the differential diagnosis of any episode of transient amnesia, it will remind clinicians to consider, and hence ask for the relevant clinical features of, migraine as a possible cause, in the same way that features of epilepsy are sought for the differential of transient epileptic amnesia. It is a more focused term than the generic "late-life migraine accompaniments", which does not appear to encompass TGA.[31] Adoption of the "migramnesia" terminology will obviously have implications both for ongoing investigation and management of these patients. High-quality prospective studies will be needed to reach more robust conclusions to justify the new terminology.

Acknowledgement

Adapted from: Fratalia L, Larner AJ. The clinical concurrence of migraine and transient global amnesia: "Migramnesia"? https://doi.org/10.20944/preprints202401.0486.v1. Subsequently published in modified form in *Prog Neurol Psychiatry* 2024;28:e12014.

References

1. Fisher CM, Adams RD: Transient global amnesia. Trans Am Neurol Assoc. 1958;83:143–6.
2. Larner AJ. Transient global amnesia: model, mechanism, hypothesis. Cortex. 2022;149:137–47.
3. Lin KH, Chen YT, Fuh JL et al. Migraine is associated with a higher risk of transient global amnesia: a nationwide cohort study. Eur J Neurol. 2014;21:718–24.
4. Yi M, Sherzai AZ, Ani C, Shavlik D, Ghamsary M, Lazar E, Sherzai D. Strong association between migraine and transient global amnesia: a national inpatient sample analysis. J Neuropsychiatry Clin Neurosci. 2019;31:43–8.
5. International Classification of Headache Disorders 3rd edition (ICHD3; https://ichd-3.org/).

6. Hodges JR, Warlow CP. Syndromes of transient amnesia: towards a classification. A study of 153 cases. J Neurol Neurosurg Psychiatry. 1990;53:834–43.

7. Liveing E. On megrim, sick-headache, and some allied disorders: a contribution to the pathology of nerve-storms. London: J&A Churchill, 1873.

8. Moersch F. Psychic manifestations of migraine. Am J Psych. 1924;80:697–716.

9. Nielsen JM. Memory and amnesia. Los Angeles: San Lucas Press, 1958.

10. Frank G. Amnestic episodes in migraine. A contribution to the differential diagnosis of transient global amnesia (ictus amnésique) [in German]. Schweiz Arch Neurol Neurochir Psychiatr. 1976;118:253–74.

11. Sheth RD, Riggs JE, Bodensteiner JB. Acute confusional migraine: variant of transient global amnesia. Pediatr Neurol. 1995;12:129–31.

12. Larner AJ. Acute confusional migraine and transient global amnesia: variants of cognitive migraine? Int J Clin Pract. 2013;67:1066.

13. Liampas I, Siouras AS, Siokas V et al. Migraine in transient global amnesia: a meta-analysis of observational studies. J Neurol. 2022;269:184–96.

14. Olivarius BD, Jensen TS. Transient global amnesia in migraine. Headache. 1979;19:335–8.

15. Caplan L, Chedru F, Lhermitte F, Mayman C. Transient global amnesia and migraine. Neurology. 1981;31:1167–70.

16. Dupuis MM, Pierre PH, Gonsette RE. Transient global amnesia and migraine in twin sisters. J Neurol Neurosurg Psychiatry. 1987;50:816–7.

17. Maggioni F, Mainardi F, Bellamio M, Zanchin G. Transient global amnesia triggered by migraine in monozygotic twins. Headache. 2011;51:1305–8.

18. Montagna P, Cerullo A, Cortelli P. Transient global amnesia occurring as migraine aura. J Headache Pain. 2000;1:57–9.

19. Dalla Volta G, Zavarise P, Ngonga G, Agosti C, Premi E, Padovani A. Transient global amnesia as a presenting aura. Headache. 2014;54:551–2.

20. Fernandez A, Rincon F, Mazer SP, Elkind MS. Magnetic resonance imaging changes in a patient with migraine attack and transient global amnesia after cardiac catheterization. CNS Spectr. 2005;10:980–3.

21. Donnet A. Transient global amnesia triggered by migraine in a French tertiary-care center: an 11–year retrospective analysis. Headache. 2015;55:853–9.

22. Larner AJ. Transient global amnesia. From patient encounter to clinical neuroscience (2nd edition). London: Springer, 2022:139.

23. Ahn S, Kim W, Lee YS et al. Transient global amnesia: seven years of experience with diffusion-weighted imaging in an emergency department. Eur Neurol. 2011;65:123–8.

24. Higashida K, Okazaki S, Todo K et al. A multicenter study of transient global amnesia for the better detection of magnetic resonance imaging abnormalities. Eur J Neurol. 2020;27:2117–24.

25. Lennox WG, Lennox MA. Epilepsy and related disorders (2 volumes). London: J&A Churchill, 1960.

26. Belcastro V, Striano P, Kasteleijn-Nolst Trenité DG, Villa MP, Parisi PJ.

Migralepsy, 26. hemicrania epileptica, post-ictal headache and "ictal epileptic headache": a proposal for terminology and classification revision. J Headache Pain. 2011;12:289–94.

27. Larner AJ. Migralepsy explained … perhaps? Advances in Clinical Neuroscience & Rehabilitation 2021;20(4):32–3.

28. Larner AJ. Stroke as a cause of TGA? Narrative review and hypothesis. J Neurol Disord Stroke. 2022;9(1):1189.

29. Olesen J, Jorgensen MB. Leao's spreading depression in the hippocampus explains transient global amnesia. A hypothesis. Acta Neurol Scand. 1986;73:219–20.

30. Ding X, Peng D. Transient global amnesia: an electrophysiological disorder based on cortical spreading depression-transient global amnesia model. Front Hum Neurosci. 2020;14:602496.

31. Vongvaivanich K, Lertakyamanee P, Silberstein SD, Dodick DW. Late-life migraine accompaniments: a narrative review. Cephalalgia. 2015;35:894–911.

Personification

> ... to du Bois-Reymond the "instinct for personification" was exactly the problem.[1]

Macdonald Critchley (1900–1997) first described personification of paralysed limbs in hemiplegics following an initial anosognosia nearly 70 years ago. He reported personal knowledge of patients who called their hemiplegic limbs "George", "Toby", "silly Billy", "floppy Joe", "baby", "gammy", "the immovable one", "the curse", "lazy bones", and "the nuisance". He found it strange that this phenomenon had not been previously described in the literature.[2] A case of personification of a presumed functional neurological limb disability is presented.

A 30–year-old right-handed man was referred to the neurology clinic following attendance at A&E with an abrupt onset movement disorder affecting the right arm and leg. Asked what the problem was, he held up his shaking right hand and laughed, saying "This is Trevor". Present for about one month, the shaking had become less noticeable in the leg, varied from time to time, and was worse when reaching for, rather than holding on to, objects. It had occasioned the loss of his job as a graphic designer. There was no prior or family history of movement disorder, but the patient was treated for depression with paroxetine and had been investigated for joint pains with no medical explanation found. His examination showed no abnormalities, specifically no neglect, aside from a tremor of the right hand and arm which was reduced with distraction and could be entrained with contralateral fast finger movements. The patient's affect was ostensibly cheerful, jokey, and lacking in evident concern. A provisional diagnosis of psychogenic tremor was made based on the history of abrupt onset, positive entrainment, absence of finger tremor, and the history of depression and possible somatoform disorder.[3] Standard brain magnetic resonance imaging was normal and EEG showed no correlate with the shaking movement which was present throughout the recording period.

Although most of the cases of personification reported by Critchley occurred in the context of left hemiplegia, he noted at least one such case in a right-handed man with a right-sided paralysis. A number of other common features were also noted, particularly a detached attitude towards the deficit which was treated with insouciance and cheerful acceptance, reminiscent of the anosodiaphoria first characterised by Babinski.[4] These features were shared by this patient, although since there was no prior history of anosognosia it may be a false generalisation to compare this case with personification of hemiplegic limbs.

Critchley mentioned that personification might also occur in amputees with phantom limbs, as well as in hemiplegics,[2] but no previous account of personification of neurological symptoms of presumed functional origin has been identified [at time of writing, 2010]. Apparent anosognosia for a movement disorder (hemiballismus) has been described.[5] Additionally, alien hand or limb syndrome may be associated not only with a feeling of foreigness and involuntary movements but also with personification, for example as "baby Joseph"[6] or "my little buddy".[7]

The neurobiological mechanisms in the current case are unknown but presumably involve some form of dissociation or alteration of body schema, perhaps resulting from a failure to integrate neural impulses initiating motor action with those from sensory feedback, thus leading to a sense of limb foreigness or otherness sufficient to mandate a naming process indicative of non-self. This might be conceptualised as "disentanglement between thought and action" or as a "pathology of sensory input", explanations implicated in other conditions such as perceptual distortions (Alice in Wonderland syndrome, phantom limbs in amputees, supernumerary limbs) and involuntary motor disorders (alien limb syndrome).

Acknowledgement

Adapted and extended from: Larner AJ. Critchley revisited: personification of a neurologically dysfunctional limb. *Adv Clin Neurosci Rehabil* 2010;10(2):28.

References

1. Finkelstein G. *Emil du Bois-Reymond. Neuroscience, self, and society in nineteenth-century Germany.* Cambridge: MIT Press, 2013:262.
2. Critchley M. Personification of paralysed limbs in hemiplegics. BMJ 1955;ii:284–6.
3. Bhatia KP, Schneider SA. Psychogenic tremor and related disorders. J Neurol 2007;254:569–74.
4. Babinski JM. Contribution a l'etude des troubles mentaux dans l'hemiplegique organique cerebrale (anosognosie). Revue Neurologique 1914;27:845–8.
5. Weinstein EA, Kahn RL. The syndrome of anosognosia. Arch Neurol Psychiatry 1950;64:772–91.
6. Doody RS, Jankovic J. The alien hand and related signs. J Neurol Neurosurg Psychiatry 1992;55:806–10.
7. Groom KN, Ng WK, Kevorkian G, Levy JK. Ego-syntonic alien hand syndrome after right posterior cerebral artery stroke. Arch Phys Med Rehabil 1999;80:162–5.

Pisa syndrome

Describing the tonic spasms of tetanus, William Gowers (1845–1915) noted that:

> Opisthotonic spasm is the rule, to which the exceptions are few. Rarely the trunk is bent forwards, from predominant cramp in the abdominal muscles and other flexors of the spine – "emprosthotonos". Still more rarely there is slight lateral flexion, "pleurotothonos", or the trunk and neck are rigid in a straight line, "orthotonos".[1]

Of the abnormal postures of the trunk, opisthotonos is perhaps the most familiar, consisting of arching of the back and extension of the limbs such that the body may be supported just on the head and ankles (*arc de cercle*). An example occurs in the novel *Hard Cash* (1863; Chapter XV) by Charles Reade. Mrs Maxley says her husband is dying in torment and the symptoms she reports are thought to indicate "lockjaw". Dr Sampson finds Maxley thus:

> His body was drawn up by the middle into an arch, and nothing touched the bed but the head and the heels; the toes were turned back in the most extraordinary contortion, and the teeth set by the rigor of the convulsion, and in the man's white face and fixed eyes were the horror and anxiety, that so often show themselves when the body feels itself in the grip of Death.

Sampson's diagnosis is not tetanus but strychnine poisoning (Maxley, a gardener, had previously asked him for poison to kill a mouse), and for treatment:

> He drenched his handkerchief with chloroform, sprang upon the patient like a mountain cat and chloroformed him with all his might.

Interestingly Sampson had used the same agent, a puff of chloroform, to treat Mrs Maxley's angina.

Emprosthotonos consists of flexion of the head on the trunk and the trunk on the knees, a bowed posture, sometimes with flexion of the limbs. Pleurothotonos describes lateral flexion of the trunk due to spasm in paraspinal musculature. This leaning posture has been likened to the predicament of Pisa's famous Leaning Tower, hence "Pisa syndrome".

Pisa syndrome is a consequence of dystonia of truncal musculature, characterised by twisting and bending of the upper thorax to one side, with involuntary flexion of the neck and head. Tilting symptoms occurring bilaterally may be labelled as "metronome Pisa syndrome". It may be seen in extrapyramidal disorders such as Parkinson's disease and multiple system atrophy, or as a rare extrapyramidal side effect caused by neuroleptic medications, or by cholinesterase inhibitors in Alzheimer's disease patients. Hence some form of cholinergic-dopaminergic imbalance would seem to be involved in pathogenesis.

When was the term "Pisa syndrome" introduced? The earliest record in PubMed is an article in Norwegian by Reinertsen published in 1975.[2] However, in 1972 Ekbom et al. had reported from Sweden on three cases of truncal dystonia in "elderly women with presenile dementia" as an adverse effect of butyrophenone neuroleptic medications and called the tonic flexion to one side with slight rotation "Pisa syndrome".[3] The earliest cases reported in a UK journal, although in paper from Canada, did not appear until 1985.[4]

There is now a sizeable literature on Pisa syndrome, around 200 papers on PubMed. More than 10 degrees of constant lateral curvature of the spine when upright is a suggested diagnostic criterion.[5] Of note in this context, the Leaning Tower of Pisa leans at an angle of 3.97 degrees, and at its maximum prior to remedial engineering work it was 5.5 degrees, so the Tower does not suffer from the syndrome named after it!

Acknowledgement

Unpublished manuscript, September 2024.

References

1. Gowers WR. *Manual of diseases of the nervous system* (Volume 2; 2nd edition). London: J&A Churchill, 1893: 682.
2. Reinertsen AM. Pisa syndrome. Posture disorder in elderly patients as a side effect of treatment with neuroleptics [Article in Norwegian]. *Tidsskr Nor Laegeforen* 1975; 95: 1212–5.
3. Ekbom K, Lindholm H, Ljungberg L. New dystonic syndrome associated with butyrophenone therapy. *Zeitschrift for Neurologie* 1972; 202: 94–103.
4. Yassa R. The Pisa syndrome: a report of two cases. *Br J Psychiatry* 1985; 146: 93–95.
5. Rissardo JP, Vora NM, Danaf N, Ramesh S, Shariff S, Caprara ALF. Pisa syndrome secondary to drugs: a scope review. *Geriatrics* 2024; 9(4): 100.

Romberg and his sign(s)

Few neurologists will be unfamiliar with referral letters stating that the patient has "Rhomberg's sign" or some "mild rhombergism" (capitalisation variable), a particularly irritating misnomer for the pedants amongst us. So, who was "Rhomberg," and what did he describe?

The neurologist: a brief biography[1,2,3]

Of course, all neurologists know (or should know) that the eponymous clinician is in fact Romberg, specifically Moritz Heinrich Romberg (1795–1873). Born in Saxony in 1795, he studied in Berlin and Vienna before pursuing his career in Berlin at the Charité Universitätsmedizin from 1820 until his retirement in 1867.

He has been described as one of the founders of neurology, principally on account of his book, *Lehrbuch der Nervenkrankheiten des Menschen*, published between 1840 and 1846. This has been characterised as the first formal treatise on diseases of the nervous system, which aimed to link pathology and physiology systematically. Therein, Romberg gave one of the enduring accounts of tabes dorsalis and described the pupillary findings in tertiary syphilis (before the eponymous Argyll Robertson). Elsewhere he gave a classic description of achondroplasia, and published on diverse medical and surgical topics, co-authoring papers with his nephew Eduard Heinrich Henoch.[4]

Eponymous signs[3,5,6]

Romberg is surely best known for his sign, or signs: static, sharpened, psychogenic, and dynamic variants of Romberg's sign have been described, although only the first of these originates with Romberg himself.

His particular contribution was to develop a clinically elicited neurological sign based on the observation that eye closure in patients with tabes dorsalis resulted in a tendency to sway and fall. Others had also observed this phenomenon before Romberg, such as Marshall Hall and Bernardus Brach, but not developed it for use as a sign.

Hence, Romberg's sign, or Rombergism, is adjudged present (or positive) when there is a dramatic increase in unsteadiness, sometimes with falls, after eye closure when a patient is standing comfortably. According to Goetz et al.,[7] Charcot "coined the eponym, "Romberg sign" to bring attention to a special clinical feature of tabetic patients described by Romberg," specifically their reliance on visual cues to keep their balance.

This is sometimes known as the static Romberg's test, in contrast to dynamic Romberg's test (*vide infra*). When performing the test, before asking the patient to close his or her eyes, it is necessary to position ones arms in such a way as to be able to catch the patient should they begin to fall. Patients may fall forward immediately on eye closure ("sink sign").

These phenomena result from sensory ataxia *i.e.* loss of proprioception from the feet, which occurs most commonly with posterior column spinal cord disease, not limited to patients with tabes dorsalis, in whom Romberg originally described his sign, but which may also occur in other forms of deafferentation.

There is no standardized method of "how to do it" (i.e. operationalisation of the sign), for example whether the feet should be positioned together or apart; whether the feet should be positioned heel to toe, so-called "sharpened Romberg's sign" (narrowing the standing base); whether or not shoes should be worn; the duration of observation; and how much sway indicates a positive sign.

Posturography is an attempt to quantify the Romberg test. Additionally, a "modified Romberg Test of Standing Balance on Firm and Compliant Support Surfaces" has been described,[8] with four test conditions (eyes open/closed; surface firm/compliant) ranked from 1 to 4, to try to dissect out the specific impairment of sensory input:

Test condition	Description	Sensory inputs
1	Eyes open, firm surface	Visual, proprioceptive, vestibular
2	Eyes closed, firm surface	Proprioceptive, vestibular
3	Eyes open, compliant surface	Visual, vestibular
4	Eyes closed, compliant surface	Vestibular only

Note that test condition 2 most closely approximates the usual clinical Romberg test.

A modest increase in sway on closing the eyes may be seen in normal subjects, and in patients with cerebellar ataxia, frontal lobe ataxia, and vestibular disorders (toward the side of the involved ear); on occasion these too may produce an increase in sway sufficient to cause falls. Hence, Romberg's test is not specific.

Large amplitude sway without falling, due to the patient clutching hold of furniture or the neurologist, has been labelled "psychogenic Romberg's sign", an indicator of functional stance impairment.

It has been argued that Romberg's sign is neither highly sensitive nor specific (at time of writing no dedicated test accuracy study has been reported) and, because of the risk of falling, should be abandoned in favour of testing proprioception at the big toe.[9]

Heel-toe or tandem walking, walking along a straight line by putting one foot directly in front of the other, heel to toe, as on a tight-rope, is sometimes known as the "dynamic Romberg's test". Impairment in this test may be a consequence of ataxia of either cerebellar or sensory origin.

Pryse-Phillips also lists "Romberg's spasm" as a form of masticatory spasm of unknown cause, probably dystonic.[10]

Eponymous syndromes

Romberg's name is recorded (second) in at least two syndromes, both somewhat esoteric.

Parry-Romberg syndrome is progressive hemifacial atrophy due to loss of subcutaneous tissues.[11,12] In addition to the cosmetic features, ipsilateral intracerebral abnormalities may also occur, producing neurological features such as migraine, facial pain, focal seizures, hemiparesis, hemianopia, and cognitive impairment. The condition was first described by the English physician Caleb Hillier Parry (1755–1822) in the posthumously published *Collections from the unpublished medical writings of the late Caleb Hillier Parry MD FRS* (1825; volume I, p.478–80). Romberg's account appeared over 20 years later, in 1846.

The Howship-Romberg syndrome[13] or phenomenon (widely and incorrectly referred to as a sign[14,15]) is pain or paraesthesia in the hip or groin radiating along the antero-medial thigh to the knee provoked by extension, abduction and medial rotation of the lower limb (and thus an inability to adduct the thigh) due to irritation/compression of the obturator nerve by an obturator hernia. The association of small bowel obstruction and the Howship-Romberg phenomenon is recognized amongst general surgeons to be pathognomonic of an incarcerated obturator hernia. The condition was originally described by the English surgeon John Howship (1781–1841), whilst working at St George's Hospital (Lanesborough House, Hyde Park Corner, London), around 1840.

It is likely that few neurologists will encounter either of these syndromes during their careers.

So why the confusion?

Why confuse "Romberg" with "Rhomberg"? The frequency of misspelling has been previously noted,[9] and indeed it has been claimed that this is the most misspelled eponym in neurology.[3] There are several possible explanations.

Firstly, very simplistically: homophony. In neurology, terminology incorporating the word 'rhombus' is more frequent. For example, the rhomboid muscles, major and minor, and the rhombencephalon.[16] Moreover, the letter rho (ρ) is also used as both the mathematical symbol for density and to denote Spearman's correlation coefficient.

Secondly, and probably related to the first point: familiarity. Whilst it is not suggested that rhombus is a high frequency word, Romberg is certainly lower frequency. Whereas Romberg is unlikely to be encountered prior to medical school or even, possibly, neurological training, the rhombus is a staple of even primary school geometry. Hence the latter is more familiar and this might account for the substitution. The hint of the esoteric or mathematical might link to the general unfamiliarity (or unwillingness to become familiar) with matters neurological.

Thirdly, and related to the previous point: as a medical community, clinicians have become increasingly ignorant of their history, collectively consigning many of the great neurologists of the past, including Professor Moritz Heinrich Romberg, to obscurity. Although, as shown by the preceding brief biography, a case can be made for including him in the neurological pantheon, he is not well known, or well-served by eponymous association, even though his textbook was translated into English in 1853 by Edward Sieveking, a physician at Queen Square. Sadly, his German origin might also account for his obscurity in the Anglophone world, wherein ignorance of other languages approaches the normative (and may also account for such lapses as "L'hermitte" for "Lhermitte", and hence to references to "the hermit's sign"[17]).

For those sorry to lose "Rhomberg" from the neurological lexicon, there may be possible consolation. Necker's cube, the optical illusion, drawing or copying of which features in certain cognitive screening instruments (e.g. the various iterations of the Addenbrooke's Cognitive Examination), was in fact a rhombohedron, or what is more commonly termed a rhomboid, rather than a cube[18] in the original publication of 1832 by Louis Albert Necker (1786–1861).[19,20] As cube is to rhomboid as square is to rhombus, perhaps we should (more correctly) rename this "Necker's rhomboid".

Acknowledgement

Adapted from: Baker MR, Williams TL, Larner AJ. Rehabilitating Romberg. *Adv Clin Neurosci Rehabil* 2022;21(2):15–17.

References

1. Schiffter R. Moritz Heinrich Romberg (1795–1873). *J Neurol* 2010;257:1409–10.
2. Housman B, Bellary SS, Walters A, Mirzayan N, Tubbs RS, Loukas M. Moritz Heinrich Romberg (1795–1873): early founder of neurology. *Clin Anat* 2014;27:147–9.
3. Pearce JM. Romberg and his sign. *Eur Neurol* 2005;53:210–3.
4. Romberg MH, Henoch EH. Affection of the Heart, Thyroid Gland, and Eyeballs. *Edinb Med Surg J* 1854;81:423–7.
5. Lanska DJ, Goetz CG. Romberg's sign: development, adoption, and adaptation in the 19th century. *Neurology* 2000;55:1201–6.
6. Larner AJ. A dictionary of neurological signs (4th edition). London: Springer; 2016:287.
7. Goetz CG, Bonduelle M, Gelfand T. *Charcot. Constructing neurology.* New York: Oxford University Press, 1995:109.
8. Agrawal Y, Carey JP, Hoffman HJ, Sklare DA, Schubert MC. The modified Romberg balance test: normative data in US adults. *Otol Neurotol* 2011;32:1309–11.
9. Turner MR. Romberg's test no longer stands up. *Pract Neurol* 2016;16:316.
10. Pryse-Phillips W. *Companion to clinical neurology* (2nd edition). Oxford: Oxford University Press; 2003:832.
11. Larner AJ, Bennison DP. Some observations on the aetiology of progressive hemifacial atrophy ("Parry-Romberg syndrome"). *J Neurol Neurosurg Psychiatry* 1993;56:1035–6.
12. Stone J. Parry-Romberg syndrome. *Pract Neurol* 2006;6:185–8.
13. Anon. (222) Obturator hernia: Tube and ovary in sac. *BMJ* 1903;2(2233):E58–9 (17th October).
14. Temple DF, Miller RE. Incarcerated obturator hernia: two case reports and review of the literature. *J Natl Med Assoc* 1980;72:513–5.
15. Saeed R, Ahmed M, Lara G, Mahmoud A, Nurick H. Howship-Romberg sign and bowel obstruction: a case report. *Cureus* 2019;1:e5066.
16. Chen VS, Morrison JP, Southwell MF, Foley JF, Bolon B, Elmore SA. Histology atlas of the developing prenatal and postnatal mouse central nervous system, with emphasis on prenatal days E7.5 to E18.5. *Toxicol Pathol* 2017;45:705–44.
17. Williams TL, Bates D, Baker MR. The phenomenon of Lhermitte. *Pract Neurol* 2021;21:246–8.
18. Necker LA. Observations on some remarkable optical phaenomena [sic] seen in Switzerland; and on an optical phaenomenon [sic] which occurs on viewing a figure of a crystal or geometrical solid. *London and Edinburgh Philosophical Magazine and Journal of Science*, third series 1832;1:329–37.
19. Eyles VA. Louis Necker of Geneva and his geological map of Scotland. *Transactions of the Edinburgh Geological Society* 1948;14:93–127.
20. Wade NJ, Campbell RN, Ross HE, Lingelbach B. Necker in Scotch perspective. *Perception* 2010;39:1–4.

Vestibular paroxysmia

In his celebrated textbook *Practical Neurology*, W. Bryan Matthews (1920–2001) memorably stated that "There can be few physicians so dedicated to their art that they do not experience a slight decline in spirits on learning that their patient's complaint is of giddiness" [1]. This may now be regarded as too pessimistic, since many cases of giddiness or dizziness can be readily diagnosed and treated, such as benign paroxysmal postural vertigo with the Epley manoeuvre, and vestibular migraine.[2] Another condition, vestibular paroxysmia, is an uncommon but eminently treatable cause of dizziness which can readily be identified on the basis of clinical history and neuroimaging.

Vestibular paroxysmia describes a syndrome of spontaneous, brief (< 1min), recurrent, self-limiting attacks of vertigo. Most attacks occur spontaneously, sometimes associated with head turning, and auditory symptoms (unilateral tinnitus, hyperacusis) may be reported. Magnetic resonance brain imaging is reported to show neurovascular compression of the 8th cranial nerve in more than 95% of cases.[3] Vestibular paroxysmia is thus one of the recognised cranial nerve neurovascular compression syndromes, along with trigeminal neuralgia (5th cranial nerve), hemifacial spasm (7th), and glossopharyngeal neuralgia (9th). However, it should be noted that not all neuroradiological findings of neurovascular contact are clinically symptomatic, so the imaging is helpful only in the correct clinical context.[4]

Other structural lesions of the brainstem have on occasion been reported to masquerade as vestibular paroxysmia.

Most patients with vestibular paroxysmia respond to agents such as carbamazepine or oxcarbazepine, even in low dosages, such that this is one of the suggested diagnostic criteria.[5] Surgical microvascular decompression is reserved for medically intractable cases. Long-term prognosis appears to be favourable.[6]

Although first described under this name in the 1990s,[7] it would seem unlikely that such a dramatic syndrome had not been previously encountered, far less that it was a new occurrence. It may be that some cases were previously labelled as "Tumarkin's otolithic [or otolith] crisis". The term "otolithic catastrophe" was first used in 1936 by Alexis Tumarkin (1900–1990),[8] when working as Honorary Aurist at Bootle General Hospital in Liverpool, to describe drop attacks in Ménière's disease.[8] Although vertigo was not a feature in Tumarkin's original description,[8] otolith crisis is listed in the differential diagnoses to be considered in possible vestibular paroxysmia.[5] Tumarkin is one of Liverpool's very few eponymists in medicine or surgery.

Acknowledgement

Preliminary manuscript, some of which later appeared in: Mbizvo GK, Larner AJ. A treatable cause of dizziness: vestibular paroxysmia. *Lancet* 2023;402:e8.

References

1. Matthews WB. Practical Neurology (3rd edition). Oxford: Blackwell Scientific Publications, 1975, p.76.
2. Agarwal K, Harnett J, Mehta N, Humphries F, Kaski D. Acute vertigo: getting the diagnosis right. BMJ 2022;378:e069850.
3. Brandt T, Strupp M, Dietrich M. Vestibular paroxysmia: a treatable neurovascular cross-compression syndrome. J Neurol 2016;263(Suppl1):S90–6.
4. Haller S, Etienne L, Kovari E, Varoquaux AD, Urbach H, Becker M. Imaging of neurovascular compression syndromes: trigeminal neuralgia, hemifacial spasm, vestibular paroxysmia, and glossopharyngeal neuralgia. AJNR Am J Neuroradiol 2016;37:1384–92.
5. Strupp M, Lopez-Escamez JA, Kim JS et al. Vestibular paroxysmia: diagnostic criteria. J Vestib Res 2016;26:409–15.
6. Steinmetz K, Becker-Bense S, Strobl R, Grill E, Seelos K, Huppert D. Vestibular paroxysmia: clinical characteristics and long-term course. J Neurol 2022;269:6237–45.
7. Brandt T, Dietrich M. Vestibular paroxysmia: vascular compression of the eighth nerve? Lancet 1994;343:798–9.
8. Hood D. Obituary – Alexis Tumarkin 1900–90. Br J Audiol 1991;25:217.
9. Tumarkin A. The otolithic catastrophe: a new syndrome. BMJ 1936;i:175–7.

Miscellany

Neurological literature: movement disorders

Previous articles in this "Neurological literature" series (now conveniently collected together[1]) have focused on literary accounts or narratives of various neurological disorders, including headache, epilepsy, cognitive disorders, and sleep-related disorders. Examples of possible literary accounts of movement disorders have also been mentioned in passing in the context of the works of Charles Dickens,[2] in the Sherlock Holmes stories of Arthur Conan Doyle,[3] and in the "pre-history" of Parkinson's disease.[4] Some further examples are gathered here.

Wry neck, or torticollis, or cervical dystonia

In Muriel Spark's (1918–2006) novel *Memento mori*, Olive observes that "Guy Leet ... has been diagnosed again for his neck. It's a rare type of rheumatism, it sounds like tortoise". Alec Warner gives us the correct term: "Torticollis?". More details about Guy's affliction emerge later:

> He ... suffered from a muscular rheumatism of the neck which caused his head to be perpetually thrust forward and askew. However, he adapted his eyesight and body as best he could to these defects, looking at everything sideways and getting about ... with two sticks.
>
> Guy ... gave a smile which might have appeared sinister to one who did not realize that this was only another consequence of his neck being twisted.
>
> Guy ... looked up with his schoolboy face obliquely ...[5]

This account accurately captures the twisting movements of cervical dystonia.

Akathisia

Hilary Mantel (1952–2022) is perhaps best known for her two Booker Prize winning novels *Wolf Hall* (2009) and its sequel *Bring up the bodies* (2012). In her twenties she suffered an illness which was labelled as a mental illness leading to treatment with anti-psychotic medication, the effects of which she described in her book *Giving up the ghost* (2003):

> Do you know about akathisia? It is a condition that develops as a side-effect of anti-psychotic medication, and the cunning thing about it is that it looks, and it feels, exactly like madness. The patient paces. She is unable to stay still. She wears a look of agitation and terror. She wrings her hands; she says she is in hell.

And from the inside, how does it feel? ... No physical pain has ever matched that morning's uprush of killing fear, the hammering heart ... You choke; pressure rises inside your skull. Your hands pull at your clothing and tear at your arms. Your breathing becomes ragged. Your voice is like a bird's cry and your hands flutter like wings. You want to hurl yourself against the windows and the walls. Every fibre of your being is possessed by panic. A desperate feeling of urgency – a need to act – but to do what, and how? – throbs through your whole body, like the pulses of an electric shock.[6]

This account captures both the restlessness and inner turmoil of the condition.

Apraxia

In the short story *No one's guilty* by the Argentinian author Julio Cortázar (1914–1984), one of the character's has difficulty dressing which has been interpreted as an example of ideomotor apraxia. Other reported symptoms suggest the possibility of alien hand, dystonia, myoclonus and postural instability, together pointing to a possible diagnosis of corticobasal degeneration.[7]

Levodopa-related fluctuations

Another Argentine author, Claudia Piñeiro (born 1960), structured her 2007 novel *Elena knows* around a day in the life of a patient, the titular Elena, diagnosed with Parkinson's disease, each of the book's three sections coinciding with the timing of a levodopa pill. The narrative suggests the author was familiar with the effects of Parkinson's disease and its treatment, not least in practical issues such as the inability of the protagonist to cut her toe nails (21) and the need for "Ropes to help her stand up from different places, more bibs to catch her saliva, foam neck braces to lift her chin ... adapters for the toilet seat" (43), also the requirement "to purge herself with laxatives" because the disease "made her intestines lazy" (72).

Elena "doesn't have a timetable. Her time is measured in pills" (70). For example, sometime after her midday pill:

But time, Elena's time, has stopped. There's no more levodopa to help her move. Nothing, Elena knows. She knows she has a wait ahead of her, a few minutes until she can take the next pill and then the time it takes the medicine to dissolve and begin to move through her body. The wait, that time that is measured without clocks ... (75)

The story also captures the strain experienced by Elena's carer, her daughter, Rita, and their battles with bureaucracy to obtain entitlements.

A diagnostic challenge?

In *The Trial* by Franz Kafka (1883–1924), first published 1925, one of the individuals encountered by Josef K., one of the "characterless, anaemic young people ... officials from his bank", is Kaminer, "with his involuntary grin caused by chronic muscle spasms", who later "was there with his grin at K.'s service. It would have been inhumane to make fun of that" (Chapter 1). Involuntary muscle spasms of the face may put one in mind of a dystonia, but the absence of any mention of eye closure (blepharospasm) would seem to rule out Meige syndrome. Brueghel syndrome is a possibility, since oromandibular dystonia occurs here in isolation although the various symptoms (e.g. trismus, bruxism, spasms of jaw opening, retraction of the corners of the mouth) are perhaps not typical of a grin. Facial grimacing may be seen in tardive dyskinesia, facial tics, and hemifacial spasm, but all these seem less likely possibilities based on the sparse information given and in the context of the novel, even more so the rictus of risus sardonicus seen in tetanus.

Acknowledgements

Unpublished manuscript, 2022, 2024. I thank Dr Lauren Fratalia for introducing me to the work of Claudia Piñeiro.

References

1. Larner AJ. *Neuroliterature: Patients, doctors, diseases. Literary perspectives on disorders of the nervous system.* Gloucester: Choir Press, 2019:241–292.
2. Larner AJ. Charles Dickens *qua* neurologist. *Adv Clin Neurosci Rehabil* 2002;2(1):22.
3. Larner AJ. "Neurological literature": Sherlock Holmes and neurology. *Adv Clin Neurosci Rehabil* 2011;11(1):20,22.
4. Larner AJ. Parkinson's disease before James Parkinson. *Adv Clin Neurosci Rehabil* 2014;13(7):24–25.
5. Spark M. *Memento mori.* London: Virago, 1959 [2018]:90,185,186,196.
6. Mantel H. *Giving up the ghost.* London and New York: Fourth Estate, 2003:175–176 (cited in Wiltshire J. *Frances Burney and the doctors. Patient narratives then and now.* Cambridge: Cambridge University Press, 2002:187).
7. Merello M. Julio Cortázar quotes on normal and abnormal movements: magic realism or reality? *Mov Disord* 2006;21:1062–1065.
8. Piñeiro C. *Elena knows.* Edinburgh: Charco Press, 2007 [2021].

Neurological literature: Headache 11

The ten previous installments in this unsystematic series of cases of headache found in works of (non-medical) literature have demonstrated a preponderance of female cases.[1,2] This is perhaps to be expected since the prevalence of headache is higher in women than men in the general population. Many of the writers describing headache have also been women, prompting the question as to whether they too were headache sufferers: confirmed for Elizabeth Gaskell and Charlotte Brontë, possible for others, such as Jane Austen. I previously wondered whether, in light of the compelling descriptions of headache in her novel *Possession* (1990), A.S. Byatt might have been similarly afflicted,[2] a speculation now confirmed. Following her death in November 2023, an appreciation published in the *Guardian* newspaper referred in passing to her having "splitting migraine".[3]

An interesting case of headache afflicting a young and otherwise healthy man, an Oxford undergraduate (at Exeter College) and a rower for the University, is found in the novel *Hard Cash* (1863; Chapter I) by Charles Reade (1814–1884). Whilst this work has attracted attention because of its description of the treatment of patients in private asylums,[4] and the excoriating judgment of "Dr. Wycherley", a caricature of Dr John Conolly (1794–1866),[5,6] to my knowledge no previous comment on the additional medical material has been made (Reade had no specific medical training as far as I can ascertain).

After rowing strenuously for Oxford University at Henley, Alfred Hardie "dipped his white handkerchief into the stream, then tied it viciously round his brow, doubled himself up with his head in his hands, and rocked himself like an old woman". A friend explains Hardie's behaviour: "the bloke really has awful headaches, like a girl, …". Refusing to row again, Hardie explains himself: "Hardie of Exeter is a good man in a boat when he has not got a headache. When he has got a headache, Hardie of Exeter is not worth a straw in a boat. Hardie of Exeter has a headache now. Ergo, the university would put the said Hardie into a race, headache and all, and reduce defeat to a certainty." He then "he held his aching head over his knees, absorbed in pain".

Hardie has been observed during this time by Mrs Dodd and her daughter Julia: "The young gentleman was a stranger; but they had recognised a faithful old acquaintance at the bottom of his pantomime [tying the wetted handkerchief around his head]." They offer him their smelling salts in "a little cut-glass bottle with a gold cork" and notice that "his face showed very pale; … his eyelids were rather swollen, and his young eyes troubled and almost filmy with the pain. The ladies saw, and their gentle bosoms were touched: they had heard of him as a victorious young Apollo trampling on all difficulties of mind and body; and they saw him wan, and worn, with feminine suffering: the contrast made him doubly interesting."

"You have a sad headache, sir," said Mrs. Dodd; "oblige me by trying my salts."

" … we know what a severe headache is, and should be glad to see you sit still in the shade, and excite yourself as little as possible."

The gendering of headache in these passages is of note. It is a female thing, familiar to the ladies (they "recognised a faithful old acquaintance") but not compatible with the ideal of masculinity ("rocked himself like an old woman"; "the bloke really has awful headaches, like a girl"). Hardie, "a good man in a boat when he has not got a headache", is rendered "wan, and worn, with feminine suffering" by his headache.

Acknowledgement

Unpublished manuscript, 2024.

References

1. Larner AJ. *Neuroliterature: Patients, doctors, diseases. Literary perspectives on disorders of the nervous system.* Gloucester: Choir Press, 2019:241–292.
2. Larner AJ. *Neuroliterature 2. Biography, semiology, miscellany. Further literary perspectives on disorders of the nervous system.* Gloucester: Choir Press, 2023: 223–226.
3. Allardice L. AS Byatt: a life defined by literature. 17th Nov 2023. https://www.theguardian.com/books/2023/nov/17/as-byatt-a-life-defined-by-literature
4. Subotsky F. Hard Cash (1863), Charles Reade – psychiatrists in 19th century fiction. *Br J Psychiatry* 2009; 194: 211.
5. Scull A. A Victorian alienist: John Conolly, FRCP, DCL (1794–1866). In: Bynum WF, Shepherd M, Porter R (eds.). *The anatomy of madness. Essays in the history of psychiatry. Volume I. People and ideas.* London: Routledge, 1985 [2004]: 103–149.
6. Bynum WF, Neve M. Hamlet on the couch. In: Bynum WF, Shepherd M, Porter R (eds.). *The anatomy of madness. Essays in the history of psychiatry. Volume I. People and ideas.* London: Routledge, 1985 [2004]: 289–303.

When and how did the ophthalmoscope reach England?

September 8th 1994 marked the one hundredth anniversary of the death (from a cerebral haemorrhage) of the German physiologist and physicist Hermann Ludwig Ferdinand von Helmholtz (1821–1894). This anniversary merited the attention of clinicians, and particularly of ophthalmologists, for Helmholtz's influence on medical practice is chiefly remembered for his invention of the ophthalmoscope. Although pre-eminent as a physicist, Helmholtz's first training was in medicine at the army medical school in Berlin, and thereafter he served as a surgeon in the Prussian army.

The invention of the ophthalmoscope, and hence the direct method of ophthalmoscopy, occurred during his subsequent tenure of the chair of physiology in Königsberg. Based on principles similar to Galileo's telescope, familiar to Helmholtz from his seminal work on physiological optics, the first report of the *Augenspiegel* ('eye mirror') was presented to the Physikalische Gesellschaft in Berlin on December 6th 1850, and published the following year.[1] This instrument, apparently designed to demonstrate to students how light is reflected from the retina, permitted physicians to observe the ocular media by transillumination through the pupil, investigation of the eye prior to this being limited to visual inspection with or without a magnifying glass. Many changes and improvements were subsequently incorporated in the ophthalmoscope to produce the instrument familiar to clinicians today.[2]

How did this German invention reach England? It is well-known that a number of clinicians championed its use in the United Kingdom, including Thomas Wharton Jones, Clifford Allbutt, John Hughlings Jackson, and William Gowers,[3] but this still leaves open the question of how the instrument arrived. A possible and perhaps surprising answer may be through the intermediacy of Helmholtz's friend and rival, the electrophysiologist Emil du Bois-Reymond (1818–1896).

In his biography of du Bois-Reymond, Gabriel Finkelstein notes that, whilst despairing of appointment to a position in Berlin, the physiologist explored the possibility of moving to England, becoming friends with Henry Bence Jones. Travelling to London in April 1852, in addition to his experimental paraphernalia he "let Bence Jones know that he had ordered two versions of Helmholtz's ophthalmoscope to show to the English medical community". Frustratingly, Finkelstein tells us no more about the fate of these two ophthalmoscopes, but du Bois-Reymond's visit did include a lecture at the Royal

Institution and he also met a wide spectrum of scientific colleagues. Interestingly, du Bois-Reymond's son Claude later became an ophthalmologist.[4]

Whatever may have happened in 1852, adoption of the ophthalmoscope in England was not rapid. Certainly Wharton Jones had little to say about the ophthalmoscope in his textbook of 1855.[3] John Ogle (1824–1905) published a paper on its use in 1860,[5] but it was not until later in the decade that Jackson[6] and Allbutt[7] were publishing on the subject, and Gowers' *Manual* did not appear until 1879.[8] In 1871 Allbutt stated that "The number of physicians who are working with the ophthalmoscope in England may, I believe, be counted on the fingers of one hand".[9] An account of use of the ophthalmoscope in the UK predating all of these is available.

In his history of the Liverpool Medical Institution (LMI), Shepherd reported that "A … discovery was brought to the notice of members when in 1857 Taylor introduced the ophthalmoscope to Liverpool".[10] According to Shepherd, Robert Hibbert Taylor (1813–1898) was Vice-President of the LMI in 1853, discussed "Electricity of Organic Function" there (possibly in the early 1840s), and was on the staff of the local Ear and Eye Institution. Shepherd's reference to the ophthalmoscope is to a paper in the *Liverpool Medico-Chirurgical Journal* in 1858, but in the (disintegrating) copy of the journal held in the LMI I found the paper in issue "No.5. January 1859", although bound with issues "No.3. January 1858" and "No.4. July 1858" and dated on the spine 1858. If this is designated as "Volume 2" of the *Liverpool Medico-Chirurgical Journal*, as per Shepherd, then it contains two sets of pages numbered 1–124. Taylor's ophthalmoscope paper is in the second set,[11] distinct from another paper by Taylor in the first set.[12]

Although Taylor discussed modifications of Helmholtz's original ophthalmoscope design, he did not say where or when he obtained his own instrument. He presented three cases "observed by myself" as well as one narrated by "a personal friend, and one who is well acquainted with diseases of the eye, and a good observer". As this case also included ophthalmoscopic observations (the friend reported that "I examined him with the Ophthalmoscope"),[11] it suggests that Taylor was not alone in using the instrument at this time. However, Taylor's use of the ophthalmoscope was not recored in his obituary in the *BMJ* in 1898.[13]

Acknowledgements

Unpublished manuscript, 7th April and October 2024; first two paragraphs adapted from Larner AJ. *Eye* 1994; 8: 717.

References

1. von Helmholtz H. *Beschreibung eines Augenspiegels zur Unter suchung der Netzhaut im lebenden Auge*. Berlin: Forstner, 1851.
2. Keeler CR. The ophthalmoscope in the lifetime of Hermann von Helmholtz. *Arch Ophthalmol* 2002; 120: 194–201.
3. Storey CE. Introducing the ophthalmoscope to British neurologists. *World Neurology* September 2016. HISTORY COLUMNIntroducing the Ophthalmoscope to British Neurologists (worldneurologyonline.com). [NB Helmholtz year of death incorrect here, given as "1924" instead of 1894].
4. Finkelstein G. *Emil du Bois-Reymond. Neuroscience, self, and society in nineteenth-century Germany*. Cambridge: MIT Press, 2013:131, 197.
5. Ogle JW. On the use of the ophthalmoscope as a help to diagnosis in diseases of the nervous system. *Medical Times and Gazette* 1860; 1: 572–574 (9th June).
6. Jackson JH. The ophthalmoscope, as an aid to the study of diseases of the brain. *Medical Times and Gazette* 1862; 2: 598–601 (12th December).
7. Allbutt TC. On the state of the optic nerves and retinae as seen in the insane. *BMJ* 1868; 1: 257 (14th March).
8. Gowers WR. *A manual and atlas of medical ophthalmoscopy*. London: J. & A. Churchill, 1879.
9. Allbutt TC. *On the use of the ophthalmoscope in diseases of the nervous system and of the kidneys and also in certain general disorders*. London: MacMillan and Co., 1871: 9.
10. Shepherd JA. *A history of the Liverpool Medical Institution*. Liverpool: Liverpool Medical Institution, 1979: 127.
11. Taylor RH. On the ophthalmoscope. *Liverpool Med Chirurg J* 1858–1859; 2 (January 1859): 50–59.
12. Taylor RH. On a form of defective vision, observed in sailors. *Liverpool Med Chirurg J* 1858–1859; 2 (January 1858): 48–53.
13. Anon. Robert Hibbert Taylor, M.D., L.R.C.S.Edin., Liverpool. *BMJ* 1898; 1: 251 (22nd January).

Elizabeth Gaskell meets science fiction: *North and South* (1854–1855) compared to Ursula Le Guin's *The Dispossessed* (1974)

At first sight, there may be little connection, obvious or subliminal, between the oeuvre of Elizabeth Gaskell and the genre of science fiction. However, reading one of the final interviews given by the author Ursula K. Le Guin (1929–2018), acknowledged to be one of the most significant science fiction writers of the 20th century, her interlocutor notes "You put in a plug for Elizabeth Gaskell recently", to which Le Guin replies "*North and South* is outstanding. *Mary Barton* makes me cry every damn time".[1] Elsewhere, Le Guin listed *Mary Barton* amongst her six "favorite timeless novels".[2] Le Guin's linking of the two so-called Manchester novels, a common literary critical approach,[3] is of note. Their themes of social and political difference and conflict are explored in many Le Guin novels, albeit often in settings far distant from Manchester.

As its title, perhaps initially suggested by Dickens, indicates, *North and South* (1854–1855) is a novel addressing polarities, and as such may have affinities with Le Guin's (1974) novel *The Dispossessed*. Asked if she had a favourite amongst her many books Le Guin replied "I think perhaps my favorite of the ones I've written is *The Dispossessed*. I put most into it. It's also the most faulty – probably for that reason – of my grown-up books".[4] Here I consider some possible thematic parallels and contrasts between these two works, which may perhaps have attracted Le Guin to *North and South*, but without wishing to imply in any way that Gaskell's work directly influenced Le Guin. (Spoiler alert: some of the details of the plot of *The Dispossessed* are discussed here.)

The respective protagonists of *North and South* and *The Dispossessed*, Margaret Hale and Shevek, have many differences – gender, age, occupation – but share a common trajectory: they both journey into the unknown and thus experience the disruption of change. Such journeys are at the core of many Le Guin novels (e.g. *Rocannon's World*, *City of Illusion*, *The Left Hand of Darkness*). Whilst Margaret travels from Helstone in Hampshire's New Forest to Milton-Northern in Darkshire, Shevek leaves his home planet of Anarres to go to the sister-planet of Urras. Whereas Margaret is obliged to make this transition because of her father's loss of religious faith, Shevek has chosen to leave, contrary to the principles of the autarky of Anarres and in the face of hostile opposition, in order to pursue his scientific goals. In doing so, both encounter a social order very different from the one they have left: industrial Milton for rural Helstone; capitalist Urras for an-archist Anarres.

Although inhabitants of the same country, Nicholas Higgins on several occasions calls Margaret a foreigner in Milton. Mr Hale notes the need to learn a different language, and Mrs Hale chastises her daughter for using "horrid Milton words", whilst Margaret recognises that "if I live in a factory town, I must speak factory language when I want it".[5] Likewise, although both Anarres and Urras are inhabited by people of the same origin ("Cetians"), the Anarresti having departed Urras two centuries earlier to develop their own society, Shevek must switch from his native language (Pravic) to the language of the Urrasti (Iotic). Linguistic relativity may be pertinent to the cognitions of the different societies. For example, in Pravic the words for work and play are the same, though distinguished from drudgery, which identity has "a strong ethical significance" for the Anarresti.[6]

On arrival in Milton, Margaret is about 19 years old and has experienced little of the world outside of Helstone and her aunt's home in London. She is largely ignorant of the ways of capital and labour, of the recurrent struggles between masters and men, in which matters she is educated by Mr Thornton and Nicholas Higgins. In particular, Thornton tells her of the unlimited power of, and the tyranny exercised by, the masters over the work people, of their "wise despotism", and Margaret experiences the exultation in the sense of power of the Milton masters when she attends the dinner at the Thorntons.[7] Shevek is welcomed to Urras as a celebrity, "the man from the Moon", lionized in the University of Ieu Eun, where he is given luxurious accommodation, for his work in physics. Shevek has known of Urras from childhood, but only indirectly, since by the Settlement of Anarres there is no direct communication between the two societies other than some trade. He has understood Urras as the "realm of iniquity", as the "ideological enemy", a society of "propertarians", of mutual aggression rather than of the mutual aid which pertains (at least notionally) on Anarres. Once on Urras, aged around 40, he finds that "all the operations of capitalism were as meaningless to him as the rites of a primitive religion." His hosts attend, apparently graciously, to all his needs, but in the hope of obtaining a new theory in physics which will give them material power over other planets. Shevek wishes to encounter the working people of Urras, which his hosts have kept him distant from, so he eventually absconds.[8]

Both protagonists become embroiled in a strike by the workers, Margaret inadvertently and Shevek willingly. Whereas the troops are too late to intervene at Marlborough Mills, Margaret's actions and injury having defused the situation and dispersed the crowd, the demonstration on Urras is brutally suppressed by the military power of the state.

Both protagonists have the opportunity to return to their places of origin.

Margaret once considered Helstone "about as perfect a place as any in the world" but her return (described in the longest chapter of the book, which was not included in the original serialisation in Dickens's *Household Words*) finds that change is everywhere and that nothing is the same, and moreover is revulsed by a local superstition of which she was apparently unaware previously.[9] Whether Shevek's return to Anarres will occasion similar disillusion, indeed whether he will survive the arrival to his home society, his departure having been vigorously opposed, is left open.

Both novels may prompt readers to ask themselves which mode of life, which choice of society, is to be preferred. The paternalistic agrarian Helstone or the industrial hierarchy of Milton? The an-archist Anarres or the capitalist Urras? Is there an ideal society, an Utopia? Speaking to Mr Bell of past and present, John Thornton states that "People can speak of Utopia much more easily than of the next day's duty".[10] One of Shevek's Urrasti hosts describes Shevek as "a damned naïve peasant from Utopia".[11] These are the only uses of the term "Utopia" in either book, to my knowledge. Although *The Dispossessed* is subtitled *An Ambiguous Utopia*, it is unclear (at least to this reader) whether the author is referring to Anarres or Urras, or even possibly both (notwithstanding the usage of the singular).

Of course, all such binaries are reductive. For, as Margaret observes, "each mode of life produces its own trials". Likewise, Nicholas Higgins opines that "North an' south have each getten their own troubles".[12] The same is evidently true of Anarres and Urras. Margaret has been described as a "troubling hybrid of south and north" and a similar conclusion may be reached about Shevek in that he fits neither society, since he wants the mutual solidarity of Anarres but he also wants to pursue his own intellectual interests which is only possible on Urras. Hence, unlike Margaret, who "crosses the border and does not return",[13] Shevek cannot remain with the Urrasti; "you the possessors are possessed. You are all in jail. Each alone, solitary, with a heap of what he owns".[14] Not only ideology but love may contribute to the decision regarding final destination: whereas Margaret finds Thornton in Milton, Shevek's partner and children have remained on Anarres.

As may hopefully be evident from this brief exposition, Le Guin may be as engaging an author as Gaskell, irrespective of what genre label ("science fiction", "fantasy") is applied to her work (labels which she herself deplored). A great author is a great author. So, just as readers of Jane Austen may be encouraged to read Le Guin,[15] I suggest the same may be true for readers of Elizabeth Gaskell.

Acknowledgements

Adapted from: Larner AJ. Elizabeth Gaskell meets science fiction. *Gaskell Society Newsletter* 2024; Issue 77: 9–13.

References

1. Streitfeld D (ed). *Ursula K. Le Guin. The last interview and other conversations.* London: Melville House (2019), 175–6.
2. *The Week,* 3rd December 2017.
3. Matus JL. Mary Barton and North and South. In: Matus JL (ed). *The Cambridge Companion to Elizabeth Gaskell.* Cambridge, Cambridge University Press (2007), 27–45.
4. Streitfeld, 36.
5. Ingham P (ed). *Elizabeth Gaskell. North and South.* London: Penguin Classics (2003 [1855]), 74,134,316,158,233. All quotes from *North and South* are taken from this edition.
6. Le Guin U. *The Dispossessed.* London: Gollancz (2002 [1974]), 9,79,223. All quotes from *The Dispossessed* are taken from this edition.
7. Ingham, 103,116,84,227,162.
8. Le Guin, 62,133,173,109.
9. Ingham, 29,384,390–1.
10. Ibid., 327.
11. Le Guin, 193.
12. Ingham, 295,300.
13. Ibid., xxiii,xviii.
14. Le Guin, 190.
15. Fowler KJ. *The Jane Austen Book Club.* London: Penguin (2005), 132,135,172,235–6 [esp. 236].

George Eliot, *Middlemarch*, and the West Riding Asylum at Wakefield

Suggested sources for the "dubious distinction of being the original of Mr Casaubon"[1] in George Eliot's *Middlemarch* include his namesake Isaac Casaubon (1559–1614) and Mark Pattison (1813–1884), an Oxford academic who wrote a biography of Isaac Casaubon.[2] Here, I venture to suggest another possible source, not only for Mr Edward Casaubon but also for his projected magnum opus, the *Key to All Mythologies*.

Godfrey Higgins (1772–1833), of Skellow Grange near Doncaster, was the author of *Anacalypsis: An Attempt to Draw Aside the Veil of the Saitic Isis or an Inquiry into the Origin of Languages, Nations and Religions*, published posthumously in 1836. The work remained unfinished at his death, the final chapter on Christianity incomplete, but the first volume included a Preface dated "May 1, 1833". Despite Higgins's assertion that "In all cases brevity ... has been my object",[3] the book ran to two volumes and nearly 1500 pages. Higgins described his work as a "key to unlock the secrets of antiquity"[4] and estimated that he had applied himself to it for "nearly ten hours daily for almost twenty years", during the first ten years of which he "found nothing that I sought for".[5]

Higgins's antiquarian studies were interrupted "for almost two years together ... in the performance of my duty as a justice of the peace, to reform some most shocking abuses in the York Lunatic Asylum".[6] As a magistrate in West Yorkshire, Higgins had committed a pauper to the Asylum in York whose neglect and ill-use came to light on his discharge in October 1813. Higgins then worked with Samuel Tuke (1784–1857) of the York Retreat, a Quaker institution for the mentally ill, entirely separate from the Asylum, where a policy of moral treatment, very different from the approach at the Asylum, was pursued. Together they sought to bring about reform of the Asylum.[7]

Higgins was subsequently instrumental in the foundation of the West Riding Pauper Lunatic Asylum at Wakefield, West Yorkshire – literally so, as he laid the foundation stone, circa 1817.[8] In the correspondence columns of the *Monthly Magazine*, he explained that Wakefield's new pauper lunatic asylum had emerged from the York scandal and had been shaped in both its location and architecture by advice from Samuel Tuke.[9] Higgins was later noted by Charles Dickens to be "one of the most indefatigable of reformers" of asylum practice.[10]

Haight suggested that, concerning potential originals for Casaubon, "the resemblance can be reduced to their having married much younger wives".[11] This is not the case for Higgins, who married in 1800, in his mid 20s. His candidacy rests on the parallels which may be detected between his *Anacalypsis* and Edward Casaubon's projected *Key to All Mythologies*.

Based on the internal evidence of the novel, *Middlemarch* is set between 1829 and 1832. Hence, Casaubon's "thirty years of preparation"[12] for writing the *Key to All Mythologies* would date to around 1800 to 1830, thus overlapping with Higgins's work of "almost twenty years" which spanned the period around 1813 to 1833. Higgins visited libraries overseas in pursuit of his material, including two visits to Rome, also the destination of Casaubon and Dorothea on their honeymoon for the purpose of the groom's library work.

Both authors published preliminary works. Higgins mentions a "small tract" on the pronunciation and meaning of Hebrew words,[13] and also "a book called the CELTIC DRUIDS, which I published in the year 1827".[14] From incidental material in *Middlemarch*, Casaubon's parerga apparently included pamphlets on "Biblical Cosmology"[15] and on the Catholic Question,[16] as well as a "tractate on the Egyptian Mysteries".[17] It is not clear whether the "pamphlets about the Early Church" which Casaubon sends to Dorothea were written by him or merely contain some of his "marginal manuscript".[18]

A number of characters, mythological and historical, and deities are common to both the *Anacalypsis* and the text of *Middlemarch*, for example: Xisuthrus; Chus or Cush; Mizraim; Baal; Cyrus; Dagon; and Thoth.[19]

More subjectively, a reading of Higgins's Preface might suggest a certain pedantry of tone reminiscent of that experienced when reading Mr Casaubon's pronouncements.

Of course, books other than *Anacalypsis* which attempt to "explain everything" might have been models for Casaubon's *Key to All Mythologies*.[20] Furthermore, Casaubon's fictional project may simply have been Eliot's rebuttal of "the peculiar German specialty of Naturphilosophie, an attempt to unify all knowledge into a single system of development"[21] which she would have known of from her familiarity with German language and culture and also through the philosophical and physiological interests of her partner, George Henry Lewes (1817–1878).

Is it possible, or plausible, that George Eliot had heard of Higgins and his *Anacalypsis*? Can any link be established between them? I find no mention of Higgins or *Anacalypsis* in either the *Quarry for Middlemarch*[22] or the transcription of Eliot's *Middlemarch* notebooks.[23] However, a connection between Eliot and Higgins, albeit indirect, may be discerned, the common link being the West Riding Pauper Lunatic Asylum in Wakefield.

To my knowledge, Eliot never visited Wakefield, although passed through it en route to Harrogate with Lewes in September 1864, reporting it to be "hideous".[24] However, another visit to Yorkshire, which may be more relevant, occurred in 1868, prior to the commencement of the writing of *Middlemarch*.[25]

It has been noted that two failed projects at lie at the heart of *Middlemarch*: Casaubon's *Key to All Mythologies* and Dr. Tertius Lydgate's work in "attempting to discover what might be called a key to all biology".[26] Medicine and doctors comprise one element of the novel.[27] One of the suggested models for Dr. Lydgate is Dr Clifford Allbutt (1836–1925).[28] According to George Henry Lewes's Journal for December 1868, he first became acquainted with Allbutt in July 1868,[29] and certainly both men attended the Annual Meeting of the British Medical Association in Oxford in early August 1868, as both their names appear in a book provided for the purpose of entering the names of members and visitors to the meeting.[30]

Eliot's correspondence shows that in September 1868 she and Lewes "stayed two days with Dr. Allbutt" in Leeds where he was developing his career as a physician. The only other information about this visit vouchsafed in Eliot's correspondence is that "Dr Bridges dined with us one day, and we had a great deal of delightful chat".[31]

One possible subject of conversation may have been Allbutt's work using the ophthalmoscope, an instrument for visually examining the internal media of the eye invented by the German physiologist Hermann von Helmholtz in 1851. Allbutt's work in ophthalmoscopy had been mentioned by Henry Acland in his Presidential Address at the BMA Oxford Meeting[32] and it may have been of some relevance to Lewes's interests in physiology. Some of Allbutt's pioneering work in ophthalmoscopy had been undertaken at the West Riding Pauper Lunatic Asylum whither he had been invited by the Medical Superintendent, James Crichton-Browne, and this material had been published in several medical journals earlier in the year.[33]

Allbutt was born in Dewsbury, only about 6 or 7 miles from Wakefield, so may have been aware of the West Riding Pauper Lunatic Asylum from his early years, long before he worked there, and may thus have been familiar with its foundation story and hence of the involvement and career of Godfrey Higgins. Perhaps Higgins may have been an item in the "delightful chat" shared by Eliot, Lewes, Allbutt and Bridges, the moreso as the latter was noted for his literary and philosophical interests.

Chat about the Asylum might have prompted discussion of a popular novel of the time which addressed, in part, the asylum question, namely Charles Reade's *Hard Cash* of 1863. Again this may have led to Higgins, since the scene in Chapter 33 in which the hero, Alfred Hardie, discovers a receptacle "filled with chains, iron belts, wrist-locks, muffles, and screw-locked hobbles" hidden there just prior to the arrival of the visiting justices may have been inspired by Higgins's actions of March 1814, when he visited the York Asylum unexpectedly early one morning and discovered four hidden cells only eight feet square and inches deep in excremental filth where thirteen old women had spent the night.[34]

In this context, it may be of note that *Middlemarch* is not devoid of references to disease of the brain causing or threatening insanity. Both "Bedlam" and "lunatics" are mentioned in the opening chapter.[35] Later, Mrs Cadwallader tells Dorothea "You will certainly go mad in that house alone" but finds a silver lining for her in the reflection that for "women who have no money, it is a sort of provision to go mad: they are taken care of then".[36] Mr Bulstrode fears that his lack of sleep is "a sign of threatening insanity" and implies that there are "signs of mental alienation" in the behaviour of John Raffles.[37]

The West Riding Pauper Lunatic Asylum is thus a factor common to both the putative Casaubon/Higgins and Lydgate/Allbutt linkages, but whether this is mere coincidence, or possibly strengthens any claim for Higgins as a source for Eliot's Casaubon and his *Key to All Mythologies*, remains an open, but intriguing, question.

Acknowledgement

Unpublished manuscript, April-August 2024. I thank Dr Mari Huws-Edwards for sharing with me her interest in all things Middlemarchian. Also Dr. Bob Adams who, when writing a history of York Asylum, independently had a similar idea: "I was fascinated to find out about his [Higgins's] life's work, 'Anacalypsis', about a universal religious belief system. I wonder if George Elliott [*sic*] used this book as a basis for Rev Casaubon's 'Key to all Mythologies' in Middemarch" (personal email communication, 22/10/2024). See also Adams RD. *Flighty, melancholic and wild: 250 years of mental health care in York.* York: Quacks Books, in preparation.

References and notes

1. Haight GS. *George Eliot: a biography.* London: Penguin, 1985: 448.
2. Nuttall AD. *Dead from the waist down. Scholars and scholarship in literature and the popular imagination.* New Haven and London: Yale University Press, 2003.
3. Higgins G. *Anacalypsis: An Attempt to Draw Aside the Veil of the Saitic Isis or an Inquiry into the Origin of Languages, Nations and Religions.* London: Longman, Rees, Orme, Brown, Green, and Longman, 1836: xiv.
4. Ibid., vi.
5. Ibid., viii.
6. Idem.
7. Digby A. *Madness, morality and medicine. A study of the York Retreat, 1796–1914.* Cambridge: Cambridge University Press, 1985: 240–242, 244.
8. Clarkson H. *Memories of Merry Wakefield. An octogenarian's recollections: being personal reminiscences, anecdotes, and impressions during the greater part of the nineteenth century.* Wakefield: W.H. Milnes, 1887: 200–201. Clarkson's memory on this point may have been mistaken.

9. Wynter R. 'Horrible dens of deception': Thomas Bakewell, Thomas Mulock and anti-asylum sentiments, c.1815–60. In: Knowles T, Trowbridge S (eds.). *Insanity and the lunatic asylum in the nineteenth century*. London: Pickering and Chatto, 2015: 16–17.

10. [Dickens C.] Things within Dr. Conolly's remembrance. *Household Words* 1857; 16 (401): 519.

11. Haight, 1985: 448.

12. Harvey WJ (ed.). *George Eliot. Middlemarch*. Harmondsworth: Penguin Books, 1965: 457. All subsequent page references to *Middlemarch* refer to this edition.

13. Higgins, 1836: viiin.

14. Ibid., viii. Capitals in original.

15. *Middlemarch*: 43.

16. Ibid., 90, 95; possibly this is also the "pamphlet for Peel", 321.

17. Ibid., 404.

18. Ibid., 61.

19. Ibid., 95 (Xisuthrus), 254 (Chus or Cush; Mizraim); 360 (Chus or Cush); 392 (Baal); 515 (Cyrus); 526 (Dagon; Thoth); 896 (Cyrus).

20. Nuttall, 2003: 56–63.

21. Finkelstein G. *Emil du Bois-Reymond. Neuroscience, self, and society in nineteenth-century Germany*. Cambridge: MIT Press, 2013: 16.

22. Kitchel AT (ed.). *Quarry for Middlemarch*. University of California Press, 1950.

23. Clark Pratt J, Neufeldt VA (eds.). *George Eliot's Middlemarch notebooks: a transcription*. Berkeley: University of California Press, 1979.

24. Haight GS (ed.). *The George Eliot letters. Volume IV 1862–1868*. New Haven: Yale University Press, 1955: 162. The "Vicar of Wakefield" does make one appearance in the novel; *Middlemarch*: 622.

25. Dorothea also makes a trip to Yorkshire, but her itinerary is undisclosed. *Middlemarch*: 736, 784.

26. Kidd C. *The world of Mr Casaubon. Britain's wars of mythography, 1700–1870*. Cambridge: Cambridge University Press, 2016: 29. One might also include Christy Garth's plan "to study all literatures"; *Middlemarch*: 616.

27. Briggs A. Middlemarch and the doctors. *Cambridge Journal* 1948; 1: 749–762.

28. Schneck JM. Tertius Lydgate in *Middlemarch* and Thomas Clifford Allbutt. *N Y State J Med* 1970; 70: 1086–1090.

29. Haight, 1955: 471n7 (citing "GHL Journal, 25 December 1868").

30. *British Medical Journal* 1868; 2: 177 (Allbutt); 178 (Lewes).

31. Haight, 1955: 474. John Henry Bridges (1832–1906) was a physician in Bradford, 1861–1869.

32. *British Medical Journal* 1868; 2: 126.

33. Allbutt TC. On the state of the optic nerves and retinae as seen in the insane. *Medico-Chirurgical Transactions* 1868; 51: 97–142. Also: *BMJ* 1868; 1: 257 (14th March); *Lancet* 1868; 1: 377–378 (21st March); *Medical Times and Gazette* 1868; 1: 328 (21st March).

34. Digby A. Changes in the asylum: the case of York, 1777–1815. *The Economic History Review* 1983; 36: 218–239 [at 239].
35. *Middlemarch*: 30, 31.
36. Ibid., 581.
37. Ibid., 733, 739.

Neuroliterature: David Ferrier (1843–1928)

Introduction

However great their achievements in clinical neurology and investigative neuroscience, however loud their acclamation by their peers, few if any neurologists become sufficiently famous (or infamous) to impinge on the wider public consciousness, certainly not to the point of becoming subjects for comment in popular fiction.

The only example that initially springs to my mind is the "Penfield mood organ" described in Philip K. Dick's (1968) novel *Do androids dream of electric sheep?* (on which the 1982 film *Blade Runner*, a very different a cultural artefact, was based), which is surely a reference to Wilder Penfield (1891–1976), whose work stimulating the cortex of awake patients with epilepsy undergoing surgery allowed him to map the functions of various regions of the brain.[1] In contrast, I am aware of three literary works which either mention by name,[2] or respond to the experimental work of,[3] David Ferrier (1843–1928), perhaps Penfield's ultimate precursor in the field of brain stimulation studies.

Background

David Ferrier first came to widespread prominence in the medical profession as a consequence of his experimental studies commenced in 1873 at the West Riding Pauper Lunatic Asylum in Wakefield, West Yorkshire.[4,5] Using faradic current to stimulate points on the cerebral cortex of various animals, he was able to evoke predictable motor responses from certain locations, emphasizing the complex goal-directed nature of the movements observed. Lesions of the same regions produced corresponding motor deficits. In his experimental studies, Ferrier was explicitly seeking to provide support for the clinical inferences on cortical localisation made by John Hughlings Jackson (1835–1911).

Ferrier's "initial publications caused an immediate sensation"[6] as did his experimental demonstrations at meetings of the British Medical Association and the British Association for the Advancement of Science in 1873. By the middle of the year, he had extended his work to monkeys, these findings later presented at the Royal Society in 1874 and 1875. His studies resulted in a monograph, *The functions of the brain*, published in 1876, and in that year he was elected a Fellow of the Royal Society.

Experimental studies such as those of Ferrier had been one of the factors prompting the development of a vocal anti-vivisection movement in the latter half of the 19th century.[7] Lobbying, particularly by the group known as the

Victoria Street Society, in which Frances Power Cobbe (1822–1904) was a prominent member, lead to the passing of the Cruelty to Animals Act in 1876, requiring experimenters to hold a licence issued by the Home Office in order to perform their investigations. The founding of the Physiological Society in 1876, with Ferrier one of the initial members,[8] was at least in part a response to this possible threat to the continued practice of experimental animal studies.

Despite Ferrier's findings, the issue of cortical localisation (motor centres) was still disputed by some, a matter which came to a head in a debate held at the International Medical Congress held in London in August 1881. The German physiologist Friedrich Goltz (1834–1902) demonstrated a dog without motor weakness despite what he claimed was complete destruction of the cerebral cortices, whereas Ferrier demonstrated a monkey rendered hemiplegic by a focal experimental brain lesion. Ferrier had previously been critical of, if not frankly scathing about, Goltz's experimental method ("fatal objections") in his Gulstonian Lectures of March 1878 on *The localisation of cerebral disease* delivered at the Royal College of Physicians.[9] Subsequent independent neuroanatomical studies of the experimental animals of both researchers indicated that Goltz's lesions were not as extensive as he had imagined, and hence the argument for localisation presented by Ferrier proved the scientific victor.[10,11] However, it was this public demonstration which formed the basis for Ferrier's subsequent prosecution, instigated by the anti-vivisectionists, under the Cruelty to Animals Act 1876, charged with not having an appropriate licence for performing such experiments.

The issue became a public and professional cause celebre, the British Medical Association paying Ferrier's legal fees and its lawyers representing him in court. Commentary on the trial and its ramifications appeared not only in the medical and scientific journals but also in the national and international press. Ferrier was acquitted when it became known that his colleague at King's College London, Gerald Yeo (1845–1909), had performed the surgery for which he had the appropriate licence under the Act.[12,13]

No doubt it was this legal entanglement which brought Ferrier sufficiently within the public gaze to prompt his appearance,[2] and/or the thematic use of vivisection,[3] in works of literature, some of which have subsequently been cast as "retrials"[3] of Ferrier. (Spoiler alert: In the following discussion of these three works, some plot details are made explicit.)

Wilkie Collins: *Heart and Science: A story of the present time* (1883)[14]

Written shortly after Ferrier's prosecution (the subtitle is surely significant in this respect), this work has been generally acknowledged to be as much a protest against vivisection as a novel,[2,3] although personally I find it has a pantomimic, sub-Wildean, comedic charm to it. It is known that Collins was a personal friend of Frances Power Cobbe, one of the chief anti-vivisection activists, and she is thanked in the first of the two prefaces to the novel.

Ferrier is specifically referenced in the second preface, addressed "To Readers in Particular":

> … a supposed discovery in connection with brain disease, which occupies a place of importance [in the novel], is not (as you may suspect) the fantastic product of the author's imagination. Finding his materials everywhere, he has even contrived to make use of Professor Ferrier – writing on the "Localisation of Cerebral Disease," and closing a confession of the present result of post-mortem examination of brains in these words: "We cannot even be sure, whether many of the changes discovered are the cause or the result of the Disease, or whether the two are the conjoint results of a common cause." Plenty of elbow room here for the spirit of discovery.

The source of the quotation, not specified in Collins's text, is from Ferrier's Gulstonian Lectures of 1878.[15] It appears again, in the text of the novel, near its climax, ascribed to a "celebrated physiologist" (Chapter LIX), a fair description of Ferrier by 1883.

One of the characters in the novel, Dr Nathan Benjulia, an Oxford graduate, conducts experiments on monkeys and dogs in his laboratory, which has no windows and a skylight with a white blind inside, to try to understand a brain disease (not specified). In her analysis of the novel, Laura Otis has likened Benjulia's "tickling" of the spine of one of the female characters, ten-year old Zo (Zoe), in which he claims he touches the cervical plexus (Chapter XII), to Ferrier's brain-mapping experiments, arguing that the correlation between a nervous stimulus and a specific movement in both instances suggests that Collins did read Ferrier's work.[3] But, as we all know, correlation is not causation and personally I am doubtful that Collins was able to engage in any depth with Ferrier's scientific publications rather than with the reports of them in the popular press or in anti-vivisectionist propaganda. However, Benjulia does later admit that when vivisecting a sick monkey, obtained from the zoological gardens, he thought of the child when hearing the animal's cries of suffering (Chapter XXXII).

Otis argues that the novel reiterates the central questions of Ferrier's trial, particularly the question of who is to police the performance of experimental scientific work.[3] Jessica Straley has seen the novel as Collins's reflection on the connection between scientific and literary practices, both potentially shocking and sensationalist.[16]

H.G. Wells: *The island of Doctor Moreau* (1896)[17]

Although Ferrier is not mentioned by name in Wells's novella, it has been argued that this work invokes Ferrier's research and that, like Collins, Wells enacts a "retrial" of Ferrier.[3] Certainly Wells had some scientific education, some of his teaching coming from Thomas Henry Huxley (1825–1895) in the mid-1880s at the School of Science in South Kensington (viii). It is possible that, somewhat earlier, around 1872, Ferrier was one of the demonstrators in Huxley's classes at South Kensington.[18]

The title character of the novel is a vivisector, working in isolation on a volcanic island located somewhere in the Pacific Ocean. The locked enclosure where he performs his experiments is described as a "laboratory" (97, 105). Moreau explains to the shipwreck survivor, Edward Prendick, the novel's apparent narrator, that he is committed to the "study of the plasticity of living forms" (71). Taking a gorilla, he had operated to make his "first man", finding that "it was chiefly the brain that needed moulding" (76). The resulting chimerical experimental forms, the "Beast-Folk," inhabit the island.

Prendick's disappearance is dated to 1887–8 (5–6), and whilst Moreau dates his work back 20 years (77) he and his associates have been on the island for only about ten or eleven years (11,19,75,106), when they were "howled out of the country [England]". This chronology indicates that they left London around 1876, late enough to know of Ferrier's initial publications but prior to his prosecution.

Having some scientific training himself, indeed with Huxley (29), Prendick is not unsympathetic to experimental science, yet he is revolted by the programme pursued on the island: "Had Moreau had any intelligible object I could have sympathized at least a little with him" (95).

Another possible point of neurophysiological interest in the novel is a reference to "some trick of unconscious cerebration" (34). The idea of unconscious cerebration had been developed by William Benjamin Carpenter (1813–1885), one the leading biologists of the late 19th century, for example in his *Principles of Mental Physiology* of 1874. The inclusion of this terminology cannot, I think, be accidental or attributed solely to chance wording by the author. Carpenter was a "fellow traveller" with Huxley, Huxley's "sort of man".[19]

Boddice has suggested that the Rockefeller Institute in New York, founded in 1901, was given the image of Wells's House of Pain by American antivivisectionists.[20]

Bram Stoker: *Dracula* (1897)[21]

Few novels can have achieved the cultural reach of Bram Stoker's *fin-de-siecle* novel, so no recapitulation of the plot is necessary here. However, a perhaps less well-remembered allusion occurs in the following passage:

> Men sneered at vivisection, and yet look at its results today! Why not advance science in its most difficult and vital aspect – the knowledge of the brain? Had I even the secret of one such mind – did I hold the key to the fancy of even one lunatic – I might advance my own branch of science to a pitch compared with which Burdon-Sanderson's [*sic*, with hyphen; incorrect] physiology or Ferrier's brain-knowledge would be as nothing (80).

The quotation purports to be from the diary of Dr John Seward, a clinician who, aged twenty-nine, has a lunatic asylum "all under his own care" (63). This location may be significant in view of the fact that Ferrier's original publications were, as mentioned, based on experimental researches performed at an asylum, the West Riding Pauper Lunatic Asylum, where laboratory space and experimental animals had been provided for him by Dr James Crichton-Browne, appointed Asylum superintendent at the age of twenty-six.[4,5] Seward himself does not perform any animal experimentation in the novel, and his studies of the zoophagous patient, Renfield, seem unresolved.

The passage cited is also quoted (with ellipsis) as one of the chapter epigraphs in Terrie Romano's book on John Burdon Sanderson (1828–1905) (*sic*, no hyphen; correct),[22] the nineteenth century physiologist and administrator who may have been one of Ferrier's early supporters. It may be the case that he encouraged Ferrier to move to London in 1870,[23] and that Ferrier worked for or with him at the Brown Animal Sanatory Institution in London in the early 1870s. Certainly, Burdon Sanderson communicated Ferrier's papers on cerebral stimulation in monkeys to the Royal Society in 1874 and 1875 (as Ferrier was not then FRS) and the initial meeting of what was to become the Physiological Society were held in his house in London in 1876.

In the notes to both the Penguin Classics edition and the Oxford World's Classics edition of *Dracula*, Burdon Sanderson's inappropriate hyphen is repeated, but more worryingly Oxford World's Classics misdates Ferrier's birth as 1847, rather than 1843,[24] and even more astonishingly Penguin Classics interprets "Ferrier" as James Frederick Ferrier (1808–1864), a Scottish metaphysician (444). From the context alone this attribution cannot be correct. Furthermore, even if there were any doubt, a later incident in the book surely confirms the reference to be to David Ferrier. The asylum patient Renfield is found collapsed in his cell with a right-sided paralysis (although he can still deliver an eloquent monologue, pertinent to the plot!):

The real injury was a depressed fracture of the skull, extending right up through the motor area. ... "The whole motor area seems affected. The suffusion of the brain will increase quickly, so we must trephine at once or it may be too late." (294)

The concept of a "motor area" in the brain relates directly to the clinical work of Hughlings Jackson and the experimental work of Ferrier. Stoker had written to his older brother, Thornley Stoker (1845–1912), an anatomist and surgeon who from 1876 held the chair of anatomy at the Royal College of Surgeons in Ireland, for information on the effects of skull injury and his notes for *Dracula* include a detailed response with a sketch of a man's head indicating the various effects of damage to different parts of the skull (451).

It may be noted that another neurologist is also mentioned in *Dracula*: Jean-Martin Charcot (1825–93). Seward accepts that Charcot has proved hypnotism "pretty well" (204), and its repeated use later becomes an important plot element in the pursuit of Count Dracula. With respect to Charcot, Ferrier dedicated his 1878 book of the Gulstonian lectures to him, and probably encountered him at the 1881 International Medical Congress in London, where the hemiplegic monkey demonstrated by Ferrier apparently provoked from Charcot the comment "C'est un malade!".

As in *Moreau*, there is reference in *Dracula* to unconscious cerebration,[25] used on both occasions by Seward (78, 288), once speaking of Renfield:

Unconscious cerebration was doing its work, even with the lunatic. (288)

Discussion

Ferrier's work, and more particularly its reception in lay as opposed to professional circles and discourses, influenced at least three writers in the later nineteenth century. Wilkie Collins was vigorously opposed to vivisection; Wells was tentatively in favour. Pedlar argues that Stoker is equivocal about science.[2] Then, as now, vivisection and "vivisectors" remain emotive subjects, calling forth responses not only from within but also from outside their particular fields of scientific study.

It is perhaps worthy of note that alienation, alienism, and alien intelligence lie at the heart of all these novels. The vivisectors in these novels, Benjulia and Moreau (and the term might possibly be extended to Dracula) are aliens from, and alienated from, normal society, living remotely, interacting little with the outside world and often then through the medium of others. Seward is an alienist by profession, and Prendick seeks a mental specialist on his escape from Moreau's island.

Acknowledgement

Adapted and extended from: Larner AJ. Neuroliterature: David Ferrier (1843–1928). *Adv Clin Neurosci Rehabil* 2023;22(2):20–22. At the time of writing, I was unaware of the paper by Finn & Stark (Medical science and the Cruelty to Animals Act 1876: a re-examination of anti-vivisectionism in provincial Britain. *Studies in History and Philosophy of Biological and Biomedical Sciences* 2015; 49: 12–23) which briefly (p.17) mentions all three literary works discussed here (ditto Finn, 2012:162). However, they err (p.17n43) in stating that Otis (my reference 3) "suggests that Collins and Stoker [*sic*] 're-tried' Ferrier through literature after the failed 1881 case" whereas Otis in fact examines the works by Collins and Wells but does not mention Stoker.

References

1. Larner AJ. "Neurological literature": neurophysiology. *Adv Clin Neurosci Rehabil.* 2017; 16(5): 14–15.
2. Pedlar V. Experimentation or exploitation? The investigations of David Ferrier, Dr Benjulia, and Dr Seward. *Interdiscip Sci Rev* 2003; 28: 169–174.
3. Otis L. Howled out of the Country: Wilkie Collins and H.G. Wells retry David Ferrier. In: Stiles A (ed.). *Neurology and Literature, 1860–1920.* Basingstoke: Palgrave Macmillan, 2007: 27–51.
4. Ferrier D. Experimental researches in cerebral physiology and pathology. *West Riding Lunatic Asylum Medical Reports* 1873; 3: 30–96.
5. Larner AJ. A month in the country: the sesquicentenary of David Ferrier's classical cerebral localisation researches of 1873. *J R Coll Physicians Edinb* 2023; 53: 128–131.
6. Young, RM. *Mind, brain and adaptation in the nineteenth century: cerebral localization and its biological context from Gall to Ferrier.* Oxford: Clarendon Press, 1970: 237.
7. French RD. *Antivivisection and medical science in Victorian society.* Princeton: Princeton University Press, 1975.
8. Sharpey-Schafer E. *History of the Physiological Society during its first fifty years, 1876–1926.* London: Cambridge University Press, 1927: 8.
9. Ferrier D. *The localisation of cerebral disease being the Gulstonian [sic] Lectures of the Royal College of Physicians for 1878.* London: Smith, Elder & Co., 1878: 121.
10. Phillips CG, Zeki S, Barlow HB. Localization of function in the cerebral cortex. Past, present and future. *Brain* 1984; 107: 327–361.
11. Tyler KL, Malessa R. The Goltz-Ferrier debates and the triumph of cerebral localizationist theory. *Neurology* 2000; 55: 1015–1024.
12. Op. cit., ref. 7: 200–202.
13. Bone I, Larner AJ. The trial of David Ferrier, November 1881: context, proceedings, and aftermath. *J Hist Neurosci* 2024; 33: 333–354.

14. All quotations are from: Collins W. *Heart and Science: A story of the present time*. First Rate Publishers (not dated, no pagination).
15. Op. cit., ref. 9: 6.
16. Straley J. Love and vivisection: Wilkie's Collins's experiment in *Heart and Science*. *Nineteenth-Century Literature* 2010; 65(3): 348–373.
17. All quotations and page references are from: Parrinder P (ed.). *H.G. Wells. The island of Doctor Moreau*. London: Penguin Classics, 2005.
18. O'Connor WJ. *Founders of British physiology. A biographical dictionary, 1820–1885*. Manchester and New York: Manchester University Press, 1988: 113, 191.
19. Desmond A. *Huxley: from devil's disciple to evolution's high priest*. London: Penguin, 1998: 186, 180.
20. Boddice R. *Humane professions: the defence of experimental medicine, 1876–1914*. Cambridge: Cambridge University Press, 2021: 158.
21. All quotations and page references are from: Hindle M. *Bram Stoker. Dracula*. London: Penguin Classics, 2003.
22. Romano TM. *Making medicine scientific. John Burdon Sanderson and the culture of Victorian science*. Baltimore and London: Johns Hopkins University Press, 2002:113.
23. Op. cit., ref. 18: 191.
24. Luckhurst R. *Bram Stoker. Dracula*. Oxford: Oxford World's Classics, 2011:375.
25. Op. cit., ref. 24: 374–375 correctly attributes the term. It is not referenced in the Penguin Classics edition.

David Ferrier's lectures on "Sleep and Dreaming" (1876): context and content considered

Introduction

David Ferrier (1843–1928) is chiefly remembered for his contributions to the understanding of the localisation of motor and sensory functions in the brain, based on both experimental studies and clinical observations published from the 1870s to the end of the 19th century.

It therefore comes as something of a surprise to find a record of him giving lectures on the subjects of "Sleep and Dreaming".

This record is found in the issue of the *Medical Press and Circular* of Wednesday 5th April 1876 which reported that "PROFESSOR FERRIER, of King's College, last week delivered a couple of interesting lectures on Sleep and Dreaming before a crowded audience at the London Institution" [capitals in original].[1] Were it not for this report, it seems possible that these lectures would have fallen below the historical event horizon: no mention of them has been found in existing biographical works on Ferrier, nor has any publication by Ferrier based on them been found. Thus, it seems worthwhile to examine the context and, as far as possible, the content of these lectures.

Context: David Ferrier

Ferrier graduated in medicine in Edinburgh in 1868 and worked for Professor Thomas Laycock (1812–1876) before travelling to England, working in London from 1870 onwards, where he quickly established contact with John Hughlings Jackson, another of Laycock's proteges. From 1871 Ferrier worked at King's College Hospital, initially as Assistant-Demonstrator of Practical Physiology and subsequently as Professor of Forensic Medicine in 1872. However, it was his experimental work undertaken at the laboratory of the West Riding Pauper Lunatic Asylum in Wakefield, West Yorkshire, in the Spring of 1873 which brought him to prominence in the medical profession.[2]

In a variety of animals (guinea-pigs, rabbits, cats, dogs) under chloroform anaesthesia, Ferrier used faradic stimulation of the exposed cerebral cortex to demonstrate that certain muscular movements were produced on the application of the electrode to certain portions of the brain, areas which he defined as cortical centres. He gave demonstrations of his experimental findings at the 1873 annual meetings of the British Medical Association held in London and the British Association for the Advancement of Science held in Bradford, garnering much notice and comment in the medical journals, and also at the medical *conversazione* held at the West Riding Asylum in November 1873. He extended the work to monkeys, experiments undertaken in London with funding from the Royal Society and subsequently published in their journals in 1874 and 1875.

Hence by the Spring of 1876, Ferrier was a relatively well-known up-and-coming neuroscientific investigator. He was working on a monograph summarising his experimental findings, entitled *The Functions of the Brain*, to be published later in the year. A proposal for his election to the Fellowship of the Royal Society was in progress, culminating in his election on 1st June 1876. He was also Assistant-Physician to King's College Hospital, as well as building his income from private practice. Domestically, he was recently married and had a daughter under one year of age. Hence it was at a very busy period in his life that he delivered his lectures on "Sleep and Dreaming" to the audience at the London Institution.

Context: The London Institution

The London Institution, not to be confused with the Royal Institution, was founded in 1805, moving to a purpose-built home in Finsbury Circus in 1819. It was at this time that a tradition of hosting scientific lectures commenced, whereas research in the in-house laboratory only began in 1841. Lectures covered a wide range of topics in natural history, including chemistry, physics, and geology, as well as biology, with audiences sometimes numbering several hundred.[3,4] Ferrier had first lectured at the London Institution in the 1874–5 session, delivering two afternoon lectures on "The Functions of the Brain". He returned in the 1875–6 session for the two afternoon lectures on "Sleep and Dreaming".

How lecturers were engaged by the London Institution's managers is unknown, but it seems likely that arrangements were made through personal contacts.[4] In this context, it is of note that one of the lecturers in the 1872–3 session was William Rutherford (1839–1899), Professor of Physiology at King's College, London, hence a colleague of Ferrier. Rutherford returned to Edinburgh in 1874, so might possibly have recommended Ferrier to replace him as a lecturer. Another possible source of recommendation might have been William Carpenter (1813–1885), who had been lecturing on various physiological topics at the London Institution since the 1850s (including on the physiology of the nervous system in 1852–3), and who had shared a plat-form with Ferrier at the annual medical *conversazione* at the West Riding Asylum held in November 1873, specifically to address Ferrier's initial findings on cortical localisation (Ferrier gave a further experimental demonstration of his work on the same evening).

The Hunterian Society was "accommodated" (library, meetings) at the London Institution for many years from the mid-1860s, in which context Hughlings Jackson delivered a lecture there ("in the large lecture theatre") on 24th February 1892 on the subject of "Neurological Fragments" (noted in *BMJ* 1892;1:350).

Context: 19th century ideas on the neurobiology of sleep

Ferrier delivered his lectures at the beginning of the final quarter of the 19th century, a time when sleep medicine as a discipline did not exist. In this context, William Dement has evocatively described this period as "prehistoric" and averred that a "passive process theory" prevailed, meaning that most clinicians subscribed to the view that sleep was a consequence of inadequate sensory stimuli to maintain the waking state.[5]

Kohlschütter's 1863 study applying various acoustic stimuli to assess depth of sleep is sometimes credited as the first experimental evaluation of sleep.[6] In 1877, Richard Caton, in his "observations on the relation of the electric currents to the function of the brain", noted that "a variation of the current frequently occurred when the rabbit awoke from sleep",[7] although it was to be more than 50 years until Hans Berger (1873–1941) developed electroencephalography as a clinical investigation which might be applied to the investigation of sleep. Overall, the 19th century has been broadly characterised as the "age of sleep theories",[8] rather than an epoch in which much was learned about the neurobiology of sleep, although clinical descriptions of some sleep-related disorders were produced during this century.[6]

Ferrier had taken his cue for his experimental studies on cerebral localisation from the clinical studies and inferences made by Hughlings Jackson. The latter had published on epilepsy, aphasia, and chorea, but had little to say about sleep and dreaming. In an 1874 editorial on drunkeness he had stated that "Dreaming is a physiological insanity",[9] but it was not until the 1890s that he returned to the subject, although he did have an interest in "dreamy states" in relation to epileptic seizures.

Content: Ferrier's ideas on sleep and dreaming

Ferrier's lectures were "delivered … before a crowded audience" at the London Institution in late March or early April 1876. Much of the published account was devoted to the first lecture, on sleep; only a brief concluding paragraph addressed the lecture on dreaming.[1]

Ferrier's aim, stated at the outset of his first lecture, was to "reduce the phenomena of sleep and dreaming to the operations of strict natural laws". His formulation was that all activity or work in the body entailed a balance between processes of waste and repair, respectively expending and replenishing body stores of energy, with waste prevailing in periods of activity and repair in periods of rest. He illustrated these principles with examples: the application of heat to an amoeba, or repetitive stimuli delivered to the frog nerve-muscle preparation, both leading to activity followed by exhaustion. Organs apparently in constant action, such as the heart and lungs, were in fact able to rest or "sleep" during the rhythmical periods of inaction between their phases of action.

Coming to the brain, "the organ of conscious activity", Ferrier's view was that since it was kept in constant action during the day it required a prolonged period of relaxation and "repair of the brain waste conditioned by all thought, solution, &c.". This "rest of the brain was sleep *par excellence*" which also afforded repair in the body generally. Ferrier also noted that active exertion of any organ, including the brain, resulted in an increase in its circulation through the reflex dilatation of local blood vessels, this hyperaemia contrasting with the "anaemia" of the brain during sleep. By drawing blood away from the brain, digestion promoted sleep, whereas sleep was prevented by "whatever tends to keep up the activity of the brain cells and the circulation".

The account of Ferrier's second lecture, on dreaming, was merely perfunctory. Ferrier's view was reported to be that "dreams are but the results of the partial activity of the brain, when the organs of attention are at rest". Evidently, the reporter allowed his personal views to intrude here, based on "the very common power of waking at any given time a person wills the night before", an observation he held to be at odds with Ferrier's argument that the "functions of attention are those which take the most profound rest".

Discussion

Only a second-hand account of Ferrier's lectures written by an anonymous reporter for the *Medical Press and Circular* is available, rather than Ferrier's own lecture notes, so care must be exercised in attempting any assessment of Ferrier's thoughts on the subjects of sleep and dreaming. From the very limited material at our disposal, Ferrier does not appear to have presented any first-hand experimental data, nor formulated any testable hypotheses, rather he gave a summary of some existing ideas.

Ferrier reportedly cited some experimental work in his lectures: studies by Max von Pettenkofer (1818–1901) and his colleague Voit allegedly showing that more oxygen was given off than taken in during the day, excess oxygen being stored up during sleep; and studies by "Durham, Hammond, &c." on reduced brain blood flow during sleep. These latter two citations indicate that Ferrier had some familiarity with current thinking on sleep.

Arthur Edward Durham (1834–1895),[10,11] Surgeon to Guy's Hospital, London, 1861–1894, had published on the physiology of sleep in 1860. Trephining the skull of anaesthetised dogs (rabbits proved less satisfactory), he had observed the blood vessels of the pia mater with both the naked eye and with a lens and found that as chloroform anaesthesia lightened and sleep ensued the brain became paler and the vessels less distended, changed reversed when the animal was roused. To obviate any changes in air pressure as the cause of his findings he inserted accurately fitting watch-glasses in place of the removed portions of bone and rendered them air-tight with inspissated Canada balsam.[12,13]

William Hammond (1828–1900), one of the founders of neurology in the USA,[14] reported similar experiments which apparently predated those of Durham although published later, prompting his observation that "the most philosophical and most carefully digested memoir upon the proximate cause of sleep, which has yet been published, is that of Mr. Durham".[15] Hammond cited Durham again in his 1869 book on "Sleep and its derangements".[16]

Did Ferrier's ideas, of sleep as a reparative process, and related in some manner to brain circulation, differ from those current in the neurological literature of the time?

Certainly ideas of brain waste and repair are found in both Durham's article[13] and in Hammond's book.[16] As for dreaming, Hammond's opinion was that "dreams are directly caused by an increased activity of the cerebral circulation over that which exists in profound sleep. This activity is probably sometimes local and at others general",[16] a view which might overlap with Ferrier's reported belief that dreams resulted from partial activity of the brain.

Did Ferrier come across the work of Durham and Hammond through his own reading, or was it brought to his attention through other means? We cannot know, but there are (at least) two suggestive pieces of evidence which may be pertinent to this question. The distinguished naturalist William Carpenter (1813–1885) gave the lecture at the 1873 West Riding Asylum medical *conversazione*, at which Ferrier also demonstrated, in which he observed that "A complete interruption of the circulation through the Brain produces immediate and complete insensibility, sensibility returning as soon as the Blood is re-admitted; while a reduction in the Blood-supply appears to be the essential condition of Sleep" [capitals in original].[17] This lecture was later published in the West Riding Asylum house journal, the *West Riding Lunatic Asylum Medical Reports*, in 1874, an issue in which Ferrier also published, as did John Milner Fothergill (1841–1888). This may have been another source of Ferrier's information about sleep. Fothergill was probably known to Ferrier in London, and he had also visited the West Riding Asylum to assess heart sounds in patients with general paralysis. In his article, he wrote:

> So it is with the brain — when functionally active, it is highly vascular; during sleep, it is pale and bloodless.
> ... the vascularity of the brain is not always the same, and experiments to prove this have been performed by Sir George Burrows, Donders, Kussmaul, and Tenner, *Arthur Durham, Hammond*, and others — experiments which show conclusively that changes can take place, and do take place, in the vascularity of the encephalon ; the brain becoming turgid during excitement, and in sleep, a period of functional quiescence, becoming pale and exsanguine [my italics].

Furthermore:

> When anaemia comes on, whether induced by sleep or by compression of the carotids ... the brain sinks down and becomes pale in colour. ... These observations, made by means of pieces of watch glass luted into the skulls of animals (rabbits and dogs), ...

The experimental details reported here (watch glass; rabbits and dogs) exactly correspond to Durham's methodology. Moreover, again echoing Durham:

> During sleep, we have every reason to believe, the actual nutrition of the brain is conducted; the more highly vascular condition of waking being associated with the functional activity of the brain. The slower current of the sleeping state favours the tissue nutrition : and consequently a condition of sleeplessness is antagonistic to or incompatible with brain nutrition and repair.[18]

Fothergill later made a further statement of what might be taken directly from Durham's conclusions:

> As sleep comes on the brain falls, becomes paler, and many of its blood-vessels that could be recognised during the waking state become indistinguishable. When consciousness returns in the act of awaking the process is reversed, the brain fills, grows ruddier, and the vessels, which were lost sight of in sleep, can again be distinguished by their enlarged calibre.[19]

Durham's work was also mentioned in passing by Charles Aldridge in the *West Riding Lunatic Asylum Medical Reports* in 1872.[20]

In a discussion of the treatment of cholera by subcutaneous injection of chloral hydrate held at the Royal Medical and Chirurgical Society in London in October 1874, at which Fothergill was present, "Dr. SANKEY referred to Mr. Durham's researches with regard to the condition of the brain in sleep. As chloral hydrate acted as a narcotic, it probably induced contraction" [capitals in original].[21] Even earlier than all of these references, Hughlings Jackson may have been aware of Durham's work, since according to Kesteven, writing in 1869:

> Dr. Hughlings Jackson, to whom we are indebted for much light thrown upon obscure questions in cerebral pathology and physiology, has confirmed the conclusions of Mr. Durham by opthalmoscopic [sic] examination of eyes during sleep.[22]

More generally, one might ask why did Ferrier deliver these lectures on sleep and dreaming? At the time he was still young, aged only 33, and developing his career as both an experimentalist and a clinician (it was not until 1880 that he was appointed at the National Hospital for the Paralysed and Epileptic at Queen Square). A certain prestige may have attached to being a lecturer at the London Institution, particularly if he had been recommended by eminent older colleagues such as Rutherford or Carpenter. It is likely that there were also fees involved. For example, in 1854, Bence Jones had informed the German physiologist Emil du Bois-Reymond that a lectureship at the London Institution would pay £10 an appearance.[23]

Accepting these as positive reasons for lecturing, Ferrier's choice of topic remains perplexing since, contrary to the 1874–5 lectures on "The Functions of the Brain", this fell outside his dedicated area of expertise. Indeed, one wonders whether Ferrier chose the subject of "Sleep and Dreaming" or whether this was requested or required of him by the London Institution's managers. Lecture topics may have been selected with a view to entertain as much as to educate the audience. In this context it may be of note that Ferrier's monograph, *The Functions of the Brain*, then in preparation for publication, contains almost nothing about either sleep or dreaming. Nor has anything relating to sleep been found in Ferrier's extensive later bibliography, either clinical or experimental.

Thus, based on the available evidence, Ferrier's lectures on "Sleep and Dreaming" appear to be no more than a brief detour in the trajectory of his clinical and research career. One wishes more information were available, but nevertheless one can agree with the parting comment of Ferrier's reporter: "There are many things in this complicated structure of man that still will puzzle and confound the most subtle reasonings of the physiologist and philosopher".[1]

Acknowledgement

Unpublished manuscript, July-August-September 2024.

References

1. Anon. Sleep and dreaming. *Med Press Circ* 1876; 21: 289–290.
2. Larner AJ. A month in the country: the sesquicentenary of David Ferrier's classical cerebral localisation researches of 1873. *J R Coll Physicians Edinb* 2023; 52: 128–131.
3. Hays JN. Science in the city: the London Institution, 1819–1840. *Br J Hist Sci* 1974; 7(2): 146–162.
4. Cutler JC. *The London Institution, 1805–1933.* Unpublished PhD thesis, University of Leicester, 1976. https://hdl.handle.net/2381/9884
5. Dement WC. The study of human sleep: a historical perspective. *Thorax* 1998; 53: S2–S7.
6. Schulz H, Salzarulo P. The development of sleep medicine: a historical sketch. *J Clin Sleep Med* 2016; 12: 1041–1052.
7. Caton R. Interim report on investigations of the electric currents of the brain. *Br Med J* 1877; Supplement: 62.
8. Thorpy MJ. History of sleep medicine. *Handb Clin Neurol* 2011; 98: 3–25.
9. [Jackson JH]. The comparative study of drunkenness. *Br Med J* 1874; 1: 685–686.
10. Anon. Arthur E. Durham, F.R.C.S.Eng., Consulting Surgeon to Guy's Hospital. *Br Med J* 1895; 1: 1067–1069.
11. Elhadd K, Larner AJ. Arthur Edward Durham (1834–1895). *J Neurol* 2024; 271: 7361–7362.
12. Durham AE. The physiology of sleep. *BMJ* 1860; 1: 548–549.
13. Durham AE. The physiology of sleep. *Guy's Hospital Reports* 1860; 6: 149–173.
14. Todman D. William Alexander Hammond (1828–1900). *J Neurol* 2008; 255: 777–778.
15. Hammond WA. *On wakefulness: with an introductory chapter of the physiology of sleep.* Philadelphia: J.B. Lippincott & Co., 1866.
16. Hammond WA. *Sleep and its derangements.* Philadelphia: J.B. Lippincott & Co., 1869.
17. Carpenter WB. On the physiological import of Dr Ferrier's experimental investigations into the functions of the brain. *West Riding Lunatic Asylum Medical Reports* 1874; 4: 1–23 [at 4].
18. Fothergill JM. Cerebral anaemia. *West Riding Lunatic Asylum Medical Reports* 1874; 4: 94–151 [at 94, 96, 97–98, 142].
19. Fothergill JM. Cerebral hyperaemia. *West Riding Lunatic Asylum Medical Reports* 1875; 5: 171–187 [at 172].
20. Aldridge C. Ophthalmoscopic observations in general paralysis, and after the

administration of certain toxic agents. *West Riding Lunatic Asylum Medical Reports* 1872; 2: 223–253 [at 232].

21. [Anon.] Royal Medical and Chirurgical Society. *BMJ* 1874; 2: 569–570 [at 570].

22. Kesteven WB. Remarks on the use of the bromides in the treatment of epilepsy and other neuroses. *J Ment Sci* 1869–1870; 15 (July 1869): 205–213 [at 212].

23. Finkelstein G. *Emil du Bois-Reymond. Neuroscience, self, and society in nineteenth-century Germany.* Cambridge: MIT Press, 2013: 155.

Winifred Holtby (1898–1935): vignettes of mental health, early 1930s

In her novel *South Riding*,[1] set in the early 1930s and published posthumously in 1936, Winifred Holtby used the responsibilities of local government to structure her portrayal of a community of individuals, her fictional location based around Yorkshire's East Riding whence Holtby herself originated. Her mother, Alice Holtby, was the first woman Alderman in the East Riding and provided the model for the fictional character of Alderman Mrs Emma Beddows.

Another character, Robert Carne, "a sporting farmer" according to the five pages of "Characters in their order of appearance" which prefaces the novel (xxi-xxvi), was based on one of Holtby's relatives who kept a racing stable and whose "aristocratic wife went mad and is now in an asylum" (xii). Likewise, the fictional Robert Carne's wife, Muriel, daughter of Lord Sedgmire, is in a private mental home in Harrogate, reportedly costing ten guineas a week (8). Although never directly encountered in the course of the novel, Muriel Carne is reported to have become mentally deranged after the birth of her daughter, Midge, and there are fears that the child may be tainted with the same affliction: "She's an unstable little thing. Heredity bad, of course." (338). When the planned marriage of Carne and her daughter had been first announced, Lady Sedgmire "had cursed and wept until her companion – a trained mental nurse – had conducted her, wailing and prophesying, from the room." (426).

Mental health is one of the themes woven into the narrative. Consistent with the remit of local government, one of the eight books comprising the novel is titled "Mental Deficiency" (305–375), in one chapter of which Alderman Mrs Beddows pays a statutory visit to the "South Riding Mental Hospital near Yarrold" (333–334) which is described as:

> … a colony of stark red buildings. Some had tall chimneys like factories; some were like Nonconformist chapels with gables and small high windows; some were like warehouses. Between them lay cinder paths and asphalt yards. To the west a large kitchen garden displayed draggled greens and wintry apple-trees as offerings to beauty.
>
> To the refined residents on the outskirts of Yarrold, these structures were an eyesore. (333)

Mrs Beddows, however, has a different point of view:

> Her judgments were not aesthetic; they were social, and they informed her that this place was good. She had known homes desolated by the ugliness of one helpless, beloved, unbiddable idiot child. She had seen the agony of spirit in men and women doomed to watch the slow dwindling of reason in those they loved. ...
>
> And her gratitude for the relief of these afflictions steeled her to make her statutory visits. She could look without flinching at the padded rooms where frenzied creatures tore wildly at the leather which at once imprisoned and protected them. She could pass from bed to bed where bodies lay, like houses tenantless, bereft of all but a strange physical survival. She could even face the more harrowing experience of refusing the pleas of the intermittently sane. (334)

A number of the patients are familiar to her, presumably based on previous visits:

> She knew now the eccentricities of the patients. ... She paid the requisite compliments to the farmer's wife, who tied up her hair with artificial flowers and thought that all the doctors were in love with her. She comforted Miss Tremaine, the saintly deaconess, who wept all day at the thought of Mortal Sin. She stroked the "cheek" of the baby held by Mother Maisie, who had killed her own child eighteen years ago in the basement scullery where it was born, and who ever since had crooned and hungered over a roll of towels cuddled in her arms. (334–335).

According to the matron, the children's wing is overcrowded and a country home for them is needed (335). Dr Flint, "Medical Officer at the County Mental Hospital" (xxvi) wants Mrs Beddows to persuade Carne to sell his failing farm cheaply for this purpose: "Air good. Grand garden, and we need a farm for the men ..." (339).

The view of Mrs Beddows, and presumably of Holtby, is later summed up:

> "As I see it, when you come to the bottom, all this local government, it's just working together – us ordinary people, against the troubles that afflict all of us – poverty, ignorance, sickness, isolation – madness." (495).

After my reading of the novel, a number of questions remained regarding these references to mental health and the arrangements for patients afflicted with psychiatric illness. Were they based on what Holtby had heard or learned from her mother? Is it pure coincidence that Mrs Beddows' maiden name is Tuke (xxi; not mentioned anywhere else in the book), a name associated with a family of reformers of mental health care in York and beyond, beginning with William Tuke who founded the York Retreat in 1796 (the name might also suggest that Mrs Beddows came from a Quaker family)? Could the depiction of the "South Riding Mental Hospital near Yarrold" be based on the Hull Borough Asylum, which had moved to Cottingham in 1883? (The map of the fictional "South Riding" (xx) seems, to my reading, to place "Yarrold" somewhere to the east of "Kingsport", the latter acknowledged to represent Hull, whereas Cottingham lies to the west of Hull.)

Some answers to these questions may be forthcoming from Marion Shaw's biography of Winifred Holtby,[2] which suggests that the novelist was writing of what she knew, both directly and indirectly. The Holtby family had moved to Cottingham in 1919 (Shaw:xii) and this was one of three areas of Yorkshire which Winifred Holtby was said to know well (Shaw:13). Alice Holtby, in her work for the East Riding County Council, was involved with mental health, setting up a new mental hospital, Broadgates, just outside Beverley (Shaw:38). On one occasion, when her mother was too tired to make a speech at a mental home, Winifred stood in for her impromptu (Shaw:41). In a letter of 25th August 1932, Winifred gave an account of a bankrupt relative whose "artistocratic wife went mad & is now in an asylum" (Shaw:238), presumably the models for Robert and Muriel Carne. An article by Winifred published in *The Listener* in 1933 described the stereotype of the spinister who "ends her life in a lunatic asylum suffering from hallucinations, melancholia, and homicidal mania" (Shaw:151).

When the Hull Borough Asylum moved from Argyle Street in Hull to De la Pole Farm at Willerby Low Road near Cottingham it was under the superintendency of Dr. John Merson (1846–ca.1936) and had been so since 1878. Reporting on the Asylum in 1889, by this time "situated six miles from Hull, at Cottingham", Daniel Hack Tuke, great-grandson of the founder of the York Retreat, stated that it was "Dr. Merson ... to whom the satisfactory state of the existing asylum is really due".[3] In his history of this institution,[4] James Bickford relates the story of "Mrs Hatfield and the great scandal" which occurred in 1922 when Merson was still Superintendent (Bickford:29–31). Councillor Mrs Hatfield, a member of the Asylum Committee who had previously voiced concerns about the Asylum to fellow Committee members, made a surprise visit to the Asylum early one morning. She found matters unsatisfactory in several areas, including bathrooms and kitchen, and later presented her report to a Council meeting rather than to the Asylum Committee. The story was apparently also taken up by a "popular weekly". A later investigation by the Board of Control largely vindicated Dr Merson and his staff, but at the time of the inquiries Mrs Merson, the Matron at the Asylum, fell ill and died, which probably hastened Dr Merson's retirement in 1924. Apparently Mrs Hatfield's concerns were:

very different from the often repeated comments of her colleagues: 'The day was glorious and the patients were enjoying themselves in the airing courts' or 'The patients seemed contented and well; only the usual complaints of detention were made'. (Bickford:31).

Whether this episode and/or these observations are pertinent to Winifred Holtby's novel is unknown, although her mother may have been aware of them from her council work, indeed may have been a visitor to the Hull Borough Asylum in her capacity of County Councillor. One may speculate that she might have related her experiences to Winifred who subsequently made use of them to inform her fictional portrayal of the "South Riding Mental Hospital" and its patients.

Acknowledgements

Adapted and much extended from: Larner AJ. Winifred Holtby (1898–1935): a mental hospital visit, early 1930s – Psychiatry in literature. *Br J Psychiatry* 2024;225:400.

References

1. Holtby W. *South Riding*. London: Virago Modern Classics, 1936 [2010]. All quotations are from this edition.
2. Shaw M. *The clear stream. A life of Winifred Holtby*. London: Virago, 1999.
3. Hack Tuke D. The past and present provision for the insane poor in Yorkshire. *BMJ* 1889; 2: 367–371 [at 369].
4. Bickford JAR. *De la Pole Hospital (1883–1983)*. Hull: Self-published, 1983.

SQ: three instances related to binary classification

What is signified by "SQ"? Three possibilities have come to my attention, all having some relation to ideas pertinent to binary classification.

The most explicit is the short story entitled "SQ" by Ursula Le Guin (1929–2018), dating from 1978.[1] The "SQ Test" of Dr Speakie "did actually literally scientifically show whether the testee was sane or insane" (362–3). "If you scored under 50 it was nice to know that you were sane, but even if you scored over 50 that was fine, too, because then you could be *helped*" in "SQ Achievement Centers" (360; italics in original). However, there is opposition to "Universal Testing", as "the Test Ban people ... accuse Dr Speakie and the Psychometric Bureau of trying to 'turn the world into a huge insane asylum'" (363). Referring to the meaning of asylum as "a place of *shelter*, a place of *care*", Dr Speakie renames the SQ Achievement Centers as "Asylums" (363; italics in original). Eventually most of the world population becomes housed in these Asylums on account of failing their SQ Test, administered quarterly, or monthly "to anyone in an executive position" (365).

No overt definition of SQ is given in the story, but from the context my own belief is that it may be "Sanity Quotient", in part because at one point Speakie states that "The preponderant inverse sanity quotient is certainly very high at the moment" (367; note that the test is negatively scored, lower scores better). I have suggested that this short story may provide an interesting illustration of the social ramifications of setting an arbitrary test threshold.[2] A distressing example from my own career in cognitive neurology was the use, bureaucratically mandated in the absence of any evidence-base, of scores on the Mini-Mental State Examination to determine eligibility or otherwise for treatment of patients with Alzheimer's disease with cholinesterase inhibitors.[3]

The second "SQ" emanates from Simon Baron-Cohen who developed the idea of a Systemizing Quotient (SQ) along with a test questionnaire which asks about level of interest in various systems which follow "if-and-then" rules, with high scores suggesting high attention to detail.[4] Baron-Cohen has suggested that such "if-and-then" rules instantiate the neural mechanisms of discovery and invention. (Disclosure: my score on the SQ-R-10, performed 27/11/2022, was 6/20, which falls within the average range for males.)

The conditional statements underpinning a decision rule may also be conceptualised as an example of "if-and-then" patterns, rules, or algorithms. Decision rules are used in some sequential diagnostic or screening testing strategies. A sequential classification decision rule, "if-and-and-and ... then," accommodating as many "and" variables as required, will increase specificity, since it has more specifiers. In the limiting "iff-and-then" case, i.e. "if-and-only-if-then," there is a single absolute specifier and hence specificity is perfect.[5]

The third "SQ" example is found in Graham Harman's philosophical explorations which led him to characterise the "quadruple object" comprising both real and sensual components, both object and qualities (RO and RQ; SO and SQ respectively).[6] On reflecting on fourfold or quadripartite structures, Harman noted that "we need to be careful not to assume that all ... quadruple structures are alike, since the only thing that fourfolds usually share in common is that they result from two separate principles of division. ... the mere existence of a fourfold structure does not prove that anything interesting has been discovered – which would require that the two axes of division are both relevant to their subject *and* somewhat surprising in their conclusions".[7] He proposed two criteria to judge the success of laying two binary oppositions crosswise:

- How well chosen are the two axes of division?
- Does a given fourfold system provide a useful account of how the four poles interrelate?[8]

These considerations of course apply to the 2x2 contingency tables, or confusion matrices, which underpin binary classification, in which "true status" (classes or instances) is cross-classified with "predicted status" (outcomes or measures). Such matrices are used to generate various outcome measures such as, for example, in test accuracy studies, sensitivity, specificity and predictive values, as well as a host of others. A more general epistemological matrix cross-classifying understanding and conscious awareness may be derived from these considerations.[9]

Acknowledgements

Unpublished manuscript, early 2024.

References

1. Le Guin UK. *The wind's twelve quarters & The compass rose*. London: Gollancz, 1978 [2015]: 359–370.
2. Larner AJ. *The 2x2 matrix. Contingency, confusion, and the metrics of binary classification* (2nd edition). London: Springer, 2024: 13.
3. Larner AJ. *Dementia in clinical practice: a neurologival perspective. Pragmatic studies in the Cognitive Function Clinic* (3rd edition). London: Springer, 2018: 301.

4. Baron-Cohen S. *The pattern seekers. A new theory of human invention.* London: Penguin, 2022: 43–44, 149–151.
5. Op. cit., ref. 2, p.217.
6. Harman G. *The quadruple object.* Winchester: Zer0 books, 2011.
7. Harman G. *Object-oriented ontology. A new theory of everything.* London: Pelican, 2018: 150–151.
8. Op. cit., ref. 6, p.80.
9. Op. cit., ref. 2, pp.242–244

Dumfries and Galloway: three neuro-history vignettes

It is perhaps to be expected that major neurological advances are developed or occur in large cities or university towns where a critical mass of clinicians and/or researchers, perhaps based in academic positions, are most likely to be found, rather than as a consequence of individuals working in isolation. Exceptions may occur, one thinks perhaps of Edward Jenner working in Gloucestershire, although he corresponded with his erstwhile mentor in London, John Hunter, about his plans. To my knowledge, the area of Dumfries and Galloway in south-west Scotland has (at least) three claims to association with major advances pertinent to the neuro-disciplines.

Anaesthesia

Most clinicians are familiar with the origin myth of ether anaesthesia and of its first successful deployment by W.T.G. Morton during surgery performed by John Collins Warren at the Massachusetts General Hospital in Boston on 16th October 1846 in the (subsequently named) Ether Dome. Likewise, the standard account of the importation of ether use to the United Kingdom is well established: Robert Liston at University College Hospital in London on 21st December 1846.[1,2] But other narratives are also available, with other claimants.

The only rapid communication between the USA and Britain at that time being by sea, the news of ether anaesthesia could only arrive in a major port. Liverpool has the claim for this first landfall, via the wooden paddle steamer *Acadia* which arrived there on 16th December 1846. Shortly thereafter, a Mr Francis Archer, surgeon to the Borough Gaol in Great Homer Street, apparently used sulphuric ether vapour whilst performing surgical operations, followed by Mr Felix Yankiewicz, a dental surgeon who exhibited an apparatus for inhaling ether vapour in January 1847.[3]

Dumfries also has a claim. Travelling on the *Acadia* was a Dr William Fraser, a native of Dumfries, who had been working as a surgeon with the Cunard Steamship Company and who had met with Morton whilst in America. At the Dumfries and Galloway Royal Infirmary on 19th December 1846, Fraser is reported to have administered sulphuric ether gas whilst Dr William Scott and Dr James McLauchlan carried out an amputation.[4] It was not however until 1872 that Scott made the claim for the priority of Dumfries over London, mentioning that he had the "information relative to the anaesthetic properties of ether from the late Dr. Fraser".[5]

In Dumfries, an inconspicuous plaque positioned low on a wall, almost at ground level, on Lindsay Terrace in Nith Bank, commemorates the event thus:

Site of
First Dumfries & Galloway
Royal Infirmary
1778 to 1873
Here the first surgical use
Of anaesthetic in Europe
Occurred on 19th December 1846

Of note, this mentions neither Fraser nor Scott, nor the anaesthetic agent used.[6]

Asylum

Besides the Infirmary, Dumfries could also boast of another medical institution, the Crichton Royal Institution. This was founded with the fortune of Dr James Crichton (1765–1823), a medical officer in the East India Company, through the philanthropy of his widow, Elizabeth Crichton (1779–1862). She had apparently decided originally to establish a University at Dumfries but the four existing Scottish Universities intervened and a Charter was refused, and a Lunatic Asylum endowed instead.[7] Here, from 1839 to 1857, William Browne (1805–1885) was enabled as superintendent to put into practice his principles for the management of the insane, as enunciated in his lectures delivered at Montrose Royal Lunatic Asylum in 1837 which were later published as *What asylums were, are, and ought to be: being the substance of five lectures delivered before the managers of the Montrose Royal Lunatic Asylum.* Browne's son James, born in 1840, grew up at Crichton Royal Institution, adopting the surname of his father's patron and patroness as his own. As James Crichton Browne, and later James Crichton-Browne, he followed in his father's footsteps in asylum medicine, most notably becoming the medical superintendent of the West Riding Pauper Lunatic Asylum at Wakefield in West Yorkshire which, under his tutelage from 1866 to 1875, was to have such a profound effect on the development of neurology in the United Kingdom, hosting David Ferrier's experimental research and publishing work by John Hughlings Jackson in its house journal.

In "Some early Crichton memories", Crichton-Browne noted that, under his father's superintendency, Crichton Royal was the venue for "the first theatrical performance ever given in a lunatic asylum" (1843) and "the first journal ever published in one" (1844).[8]

Myasthenia gravis

The symptoms of myasthenia gravis were perhaps first noted by Thomas Willis in the seventeenth century. With the panoply of therapeutic options now at the disposal of neurologists,[9] it is perhaps easily forgotten that for centuries the condition was untreatable. The first effective treatment, with physostigmine, was demonstrated by Mary Broadfoot Walker,[10-12] a native of Wigtown (now perhaps best known as "Scotland's National Book Town"). Her findings were first published in the *Lancet* in June 1934, at which time she was working at St Alfege's Hospital in Greenwich.[13] Because of the need to administer physostigmine by injection, she also tried oral neostigmine.

The word "breakthrough" is perhaps too frequently used in the context of clinical medicine, but this certainly was one, and notably emanated from a non-academic setting. Mary Walker retired to Wigtown in 1954.

Discussion

Evidently other Gallovidian, or Gallowegian,[14] contributions to medicine and surgery might be noted,[15] but those mentioned here are perhaps the most outstanding from the current perspective of posterity. Although ether has not endured as an anaesthetic agent, the discipline initiated by its discovery most certainly has. The Crichton Royal Hospital, like most of the nineteenth century asylums, is no more, but the estate still exists, including a modest statue of Elizabeth Crichton (but no memorial to William Browne, as far as I know). Although physostigmine is no longer used, oral pyridostigmine still has a role as a symptomatic treatment of myasthenia gravis.

Acknowledgements

Unpublished manuscript, 2023–4.

References

1. Stratmann L. *Chloroform. The quest for oblivion.* Stroud: Sutton Publishing, 2003: 15, 34–35.
2. Snow SJ. *Blessed days of anaesthesia. How anaesthetics changed the world.* Oxford: Oxford University Press, 2008: 24–25, 30.
3. Gray TC. Whatever happened to Felix Yankiewicz? *J R Soc Med* 1978; 71: 292–299.
4. Irving G. *Dumfries and Galloway Royal Infirmary – the first two hundred years.* Dumfries: Dumfries and Galloway Health Board, 1975: 35–40.

5. Scott W. The exhibition of ether as an anaesthetic. *Lancet* 1872; 2: 585 (October 19th).

6. Personal observation [discovered by chance], Dumfries, 12/07/2024.

7. Crichton-Browne J. *Victorian jottings from an old commonplace book.* London: Etchells and Macdonald, 1926: 35–36.

8. Easterbrook CC. *The chronicle of Crichton Royal.* Dumfries: Courier Press, 1937:23.

9. Sathasivam S, Larner AJ. Disorders of the neuromuscular junction. In: Sinclair AJ, Morley JE, Vellas B, Cesare M, Munshi M (eds.). *Pathy's principles and practice of geriatric medicine* (6th edition). Chichester: Wiley Blackwell, 2022: 709–717.

10. Pearce JMS. Mary Broadfoot Walker (1888–1974): a historic discovery in myasthenia gravis. *Eur Neurol* 2005; 53: 51–53.

11. Johnston JD. Mary Broadfoot Walker (1888–1974). *J Neurol* 2007; 254: 1306–1307.

12. McCarter SJ, Burkholder DB, Klaas JP, Martinez-Thompson JM, Boes CJ. The Mary Walker effect: Mary Broadfoot Walker. *J R Coll Physicians Edinb* 2019; 49: 255–259.

13. Walker MB. Treatment of myasthenia gravis with physostigmine. *Lancet* 1934; i: 1200–1201.

14. Crichton-Browne J. *The doctor's after thoughts.* London: Ernest Benn, 1932: 149.

15. Macintyre I. The life and work of the Dumfries surgeon James Hill (1703–1776): his contributions to the management of cancer and of head injury. *J Med Biogr* 2016; 24: 459–468.

Psychosurgery at Winwick Hospital, Warrington

Pop music fans of a certain late 1970s vintage may be familiar with the song *Teenage Lobotomy* from the 1977 album *Rocket to Russia* by the American punk band Ramones, which features the lyric:

> All the girls are in love with me
> I'm a teenage lobotomy

However, the knowledge of pertinent neuroanatomy, be it of Ramones or their neurosurgeon, leaves something to be desired:

> Guess I'll have to go and tell 'em
> That I've got no cerebellum

The development of prefrontal leucotomy, or "lobotomy", pioneered by Egas Moniz and taken to its extreme by Walter Freeman in the USA has been well documented.[1] As a chapter in the history of medicine, it is instructive of how a worthless and indeed dangerous procedure can be widely adopted. Many neurosurgeons of note took it up, including William Beecher Scoville in the USA[2] and Sir Wylie McKissock in the United Kingdom.[3]

Thousands of procedures must have been performed up until the 1950s when new psychotropic medications became available, and many leucotomised patients must have survived long term. However, in my clinical practice as a neurologist (1990s-2020s) I never encountered a survivor, although I did see one patient who had previously undergone stereotactic subcaudate tractotomy using yttrium-90 to produce the lesion, the patient presenting 30 years later with drug-induced excessive daytime somnolence.[4] This particular procedure had been performed at the Geoffrey Knight Unit, then at the Brook General Hospital in London (the unit later moved to the Maudsley Hospital).[5]

Not much is written, as far as I can ascertain, about lobotomy in the United Kingdom: Pressman exclusively addressed the American scene[1] and Berrios,[6] addressing "psychosurgery" in Britain, meaning essentially trepanation (also briefly considered by Wallis[7]), stopped his account at Moniz.

I have no clear recollection of how I heard about the possibility that leucotomies had been performed at Winwick Hospital at Warrington. This, the Fifth Lancashire County Asylum, was opened in 1902 and closed in 1997. The account of its history on the website devoted to the county asylums (www.countyasylums.co.uk) has no mention of leucotomy. The history of the asylum written by Lewis[8] has a little more information, mentioning amongst "Some of the more emotive treatments (therapies) over the years" not only ECT and insulin therapy but also "PRE FONTAL LEUCOTOMY" [*sic*; capitals in original]:

> This is a neurosurgical procedure which was employed in the postwar years although it was first carried out before the Second World War.
> It is, of course, a surgical operation usually carried out as "*a last resort*" when other treatments had been carried out without any success.
> The illnesess [*sic*] for which it was advised were those of sever [*sic*] depression or prolonged or disturbed behaviour. Many of the patients involved benefited [*sic*] to the point of being able to leave hospital. Others, whilst not reaching this goal, benefited [*sic*] in such a way as to be able to enjoy facilities within the confines of the hospital. (ref. 8, p.88; italics in original).

Amongst the observations "made by a Winwick Charge Nurse during the 1950's and 60's", it was noted under, "Major changes", that:

> As the much-practiced Leucotomy fell into disuse, a new wonder operation was done at Winwick – Pallidotomy, for the treatment of Parkinson's Disease. After one or two miraculously-impressive cases, a run of postoperative disasters led to this being abandoned. Ideas that Winwick could be a Regional Neurosurgery Unit ... were stillborn. (ref. 8, p.104).

> Treatment changes with the times and some treatments originally carried out were found wanting. Treatments such as Luecotomy [*sic*] (a severing of the frontal lobe fibres); Paladotomy [*sic*] (a surgical TX/R [*sic*] Parkinson's disease); deep insulin therapy (all stopped 1960's) preceded Electro Convulsion Therapy (E.C.T.) still playing an important role in treating predominantly depressive conditions and mania. (ref. 8, p.107).

Hence no information is given as to who performed these procedures or how many patients were involved. (One wonders if some of the pallidotomy failures might have been a consequence of operating on patients with parkinsonism as a consequence of the adverse anti-dopaminergic effects of psychotropic medications rather than idiopathic Parkinson's disease.)

At the "Winwick Hospital Remembered ..." website (www.winwickremembered.org.uk; accessed 01/06/24), the recollections of Eddie Newall ("Post-registration student nurse and staff nurse, 1969–1971") included the observation that:

> Some patients had the tell-tale indentations on either side of their forehead – signs of pre-frontal leucotomy in bygone years.

In his history of the Chester County Lunatic Asylum, known as Deva Hospital between 1953 and 1970, Stan Murphy reported that:[9]

> Pre-frontal leucotomy was performed on hundreds of patients at the Deva and other hospitals from 1947 until the late 1960s. In the 1950s Winwick Hospital became the centre where this treatment was carried out. A report dated 31/3/1957 states:
>
>> Our first leucotomy operation was in 1947 and since then 184 patients have had this brain operation. This enabled 101 patients to leave the hospital whose discharge would not otherwise have been possible. The introduction of the new tranquillising group of drugs has reduced the number of operations without replacing the need for leucotomy in some cases. For several years about 30 patients a year have had the operation. There existed a backlog of long stay patients, some of whom could benefit from leucotomy, but now most cases of these have been sifted out, and we did only 5 in 1955, and 6 in 1956. Of these 11 operations, 4 patients have gone home, recovered; 2 have improved and 5 have shown no improvement so far. (ref. 9, p.51).

It is not clear whether this information referred to cases from Winwick alone, or elsewhere (the "report dated 31/3/1957" has not been traced).

Reports on leucotomy in England and Wales published by the Board of Control in 1947 and by the Ministry of Health in 1961, covering the periods to the end of 1944 and from 1940 to 1954 respectively, recorded 1000 and between 1500–1700 procedures but gave no information as to where these operations were performed or by whom.[10,11]

Consulting the historical records specific to Winwick, some further information is forthcoming. In *Winwick Hospital Warrington. Report for the two years 1948 and 1949*, it is stated that:[12]

> during the two years under review ... 204 [patients were treated] by leucotomy. (ref. 12, p.19).

Furthermore:

> This hospital has now become a Neuro-Surgical Centre for leucotomy operations and cases are for this purpose temporarily transferred to us from Rainhill [the Second Lancashire County Asylum, at Prescot] and Upton hospitals [Chester County Lunatic Asylum was known as Upton Mental Hospital between 1948 and 1953]. The deaths occurring after leucotomy in the four years since its introduction have numbered 17 in a total series of 272, but only 11 were directly due to the operation. (ref. 12, p.19; also p.43).

This passage, along with the materials provided by Lewis[8] and by Murphy,[9] suggests two things: that leucotomy procedures were performed at Winwick Hospital at least from 1947, and possibly earlier, and were undertaken by one or more neurosurgeons. The visiting Neurosurgeons listed in the Winwick Hospital *Report* were A. Sutcliffe Kerr and R.H. Hannah. Alan Sutcliffe Kerr (1909–1977) "developed a neurosurgical service in the Emergency Medical Service Hospital at Winwick"[13] during the Second World War which transferred to the Walton Hospital in Liverpool in 1947.[14] Richard Hannah (1915–2000) was "appointed to the new unit in Liverpool in 1947".[15] Thus, if pre-frontal leuctotomy was introduced as a neurosurgical procedure at Winwick Hospital around 1945–1947, the likelihood is that these operations could only have been performed by Sutcliffe Kerr, likewise if psychosurgery was also performed in Chester.

Sutcliffe Kerr was in the United States between 1937 and 1939 on a Rockefeller scholarship, based in St. Louis, Missouri.[16] It is just possible that whilst there he may have heard of the first lobotomy procedures performed by Freeman and Watts from 1936 onwards. Sutcliffe Kerr returned to the UK before the war. Freeman and Watts monograph entitled *Psychosurgery* was published in 1942, but apparently the only shipment of the volume to Europe was torpedoed.[17]

In the context of Chester, a newspaper report from early 1949 is instructive:

> ... at an inquest at Chester today on a patient at the County Mental Hopsital, Chester.

> Mr. Alan Sutcliffe Kerr, neurosurgeon to the Liverpool hospital region, said he carried out an operation, known as pre-frontal leucotomy, on January 11.

> The patient had an epileptic attack at the beginning of the operation. When the wound was being closed, she had six further fits within seven minutes and died.[18]

At time of writing, I have found no publication from Liverpool on the subject of psychosurgery in the medical literature. Neither Sutcliffe Kerr nor Hannah appears to have been involved in the "Anglo-American Symposium on Psychosurgery, Neurophysiology and Physical Treatments in Psychiatry" held at the Royal Society of Medicine in 1949.[19]

Another possibility, albeit unlikely, is that one or more of the psychiatrists working at Winwick learned or took on the leucotomy procedure, rather than simply recommending it on clinical grounds to the neurosurgeon. (Harry Fleming, a psychiatrist at Winwick, was once reported to be involved with leucotomy: *Manchester Guardian* 2ⁿᵈ April 1968, p.6.) If so, it is difficult to see how Winwick could be described as "a Neuro-Surgical Centre". Moreover, it is difficult to imagine that any neurosurgeon would acquiesce in the idea of an untrained psychiatrist performing such invasive procedures. No visiting neurologist was listed in the Winwick Hospital *Report*, and at this time the only neurologist in the Mersey region was Dr. R.R. Hughes.

Acknowledgements

Unpublished manuscript, 2024. Thanks to staff at the Chester Record Office for help in accessing the publications by Lewis and Murphy.

References

1. Pressman JD. *Last resort. Psychosurgery and the limits of medicine.* Cambridge: Cambridge University Press, 1998.
2. Dittrich L. *Patient H.M. A story of memory, madness and family secrets.* London: Chatto & Windus, 2016 [esp. 144–156].
3. McKissock W. Rostral leucotomy. *Lancet* 1951: 2(6673): 91–94.
4. Abernethy Holland AJ, Larner AJ. Yttrium-90 implantation. *Prog Neurol Psychiatry* 2009; 13(5): 27.
5. Bridges PK, Bartlett JR, Hale AS, Poynton AM, Malizia AL, Hodgkiss AD. Psychosurgery: stereotactic subcaudate tractotomy. An indispensable treatment. *Br J Psychiatry* 1994; 165: 599–611.
6. Berrios GE. Psychosurgery in Britain and elsewhere: a conceptual history. In: Berrios GE, Freeman H (eds.) *150 years of British Psychiatry 1841–1991.* London: Royal College of Psychiatrists, 1991: 180–196.
7. Wallis J. *Investigating the body in the Victorian Asylum. Doctors, patients, and practices.* London: Palgrave Macmillan, 2017: 186–191.
8. Lewis K. *Lancaster County Asylum, Winwick. Lancashire last asylum. "A place of safety" 1897–1997.* Newton-le-Willows: Willow Printing, 1995.
9. Murphy S. *The best is yet to be. 175ᵗʰ anniversary history of the West Cheshire Hospital, with memories from the Moston and Manor hospitals.* Chester: C.C. Publishing, 2004.
10. Board of Control (England and Wales). *Pre-frontal leucotomy in 1,000 cases.* London: HMSO, 1947.
11. Tooth GC, Newton MP. *Leucotomy in England and Wales 1942–1954* (Ministry of Health Reports on Public Health and Medical Subjects No. 104). London: HMSO, 1961.
12. *Winwick Hospital Warrington. Report for the two years 1948 and 1949.*
13. *Plarr's Lives of the Fellows online*, https://livesonline.rcseng.ac.uk/biogs/E006652.htm (accessed 02/06/24).
14. Clitherow N. 1947: Neurosurgery comes to Walton Hospital. *Medical Historian (Journal of the Liverpool Medical History Society)* 2018; 28: 19–21.

15. Miles J. Richard Hannah. *BMJ* 2000; 321: 388.

16. Sedzimir CB. Obituary: Alan Sutcliffe Kerr. *Acta Neurochirurgica* 1977; 38: 173–175 [at 174].

17. Op. cit., ref. 1, p. 481n57.

18. *Liverpool Evening Express*, 16th February 1949, p.1 (Had seven fits, died. Mental patient's operation).

19. Anglo-American Symposium on psychosurgery, neurophysiology and physical treatments in psychiatry. *Proc R Soc Med* 1949; 42(Suppl).

Sherrington as Editor: *Thompson Yates (and Johnston) Laboratories Report*

As is well known, Charles Scott Sherrington (1857–1952) was the chairman of the editorial board of the *Journal of Physiology* from 1926 to 1935, only the third editor of the *Journal* after its inception in 1878, following Michael Foster (editor 1878–1906) and John Newport Langley (editor 1878–1926). Hence Sherrington presided over the 50th anniversary of the *Journal* in 1928. By this time, he was Waynflete Professor of Physiology in the University of Oxford, having arrived in Oxford from Liverpool where he had been Holt Professor of Physiology from 1895 to 1913. As reported by Liddell (1952:256), "from October 1898 he [Sherrington] was to have his share of the new Thompson-Yates [*sic*] laboratories for physiology and pathology which were very much to his liking and convenience". Sherrington's Liverpool years included his Silliman Memorial Lectures delivered at Yale in 1904 which were later published as his seminal work, *The integrative action of the nervous system*, in 1906.

The *Journal of Physiology* may have been the pinnacle of Sherrington's career as an editor, but it was not the first journal of which he held the editorship. Although a fact which may not be widely known, between 1898 and 1905 Sherrington was the co-editor of the house journal of the Thompson Yates Laboratories in Liverpool. In the years 1898 to 1902 this journal was called the *Thompson Yates Laboratories Report*, and, following further funding, from 1903 to 1905 the *Thompson Yates and Johnston Laboratories Report*. In all, seven volumes appeared. Two parts were issued each year.

To my knowledge, no previous publications have been devoted to Sherrington as editor or to the *Thompson Yates (and Johnston) Laboratories Report*.

Contents of *Thompson Yates (and Johnston) Laboratories Report* (see Table)

As announced on the title page of each volume, the journal was edited jointly by Sherrington and by Rubert Boyce, the Professor of Pathology at University College Liverpool, who also shared the facilities of the Thompson Yates Laboratories. The title page also noted that the journal appeared "with the co-operation of" a cast list of other individuals working in the Thompson Yates Laboratories, in the fields of Physiology and Chemical Physiology, Animal Histology, Pathology and Bacteriology, Comparative Pathology, Neurology, Tropical Medicine, and Hygiene. The subject matter of the journal was thus broad.

The Preface of the first volume stated that:

The Thompson Yates Laboratory Reports will be issued half-yearly, or oftener, if sufficient material is ready for publication.

They are intended to promote learning and record Research in the various branches of Physiology and Pathology, and thus to carry out the wishes of the Founders of these Schools.

Two volumes are now published. The first volume contains the account of the opening of the Laboratories in October, 1898, by Lord Lister, P.R.S., who was accompanied on that occasion by Professor Virchow and a distinguished gathering of Scientific and representative men. An address delivered before the Medical Students of University College by the Founder of the Laboratories, the Rev. SAMUEL ASHTON THOMPSON YATES, will be also found in the first volume.

In the second volume reports are given of the various departments which clearly indicate the numerous ways in which the University teaching in these schools is directly applicable to the needs of the community, including the wide sphere of our Colonies, both as regards the prevention and cure of disease at home and abroad and the advancement of Commerce.

Our best thanks are due to the Council of the Royal Society, to the Council of the Royal Medical Chirurgical Society's Transactions, and to the Editors of the 'British Medical Journal,' 'Lancet,' 'Liverpool Medical Chirurgical Journal,' 'Brain,' 'Journal of Physiology and of Pathology,' the Committee of the Liverpool School of Tropical Medicine, and the Lancashire Sea Fisheries, for kindly allowing us to reprint papers which have appeared in their journals. [capitals in original].

The dating of the journal volumes may be confusing. The first issue was dated on the title page as "1898–1899", immediately below which apperead "At the University Press of Liverpool 1900". The first issue comprised volumes 1 and 2, both dated 1898–1899, and the former included reprints of a number of papers by Sherrington and by others which had appeared in 1898 and 1899. I presume the "1898–1899" was to mark the date of opening of the Thompson Yates Laboratories, but evidently the volume was not ready for the press until 1900. Succeeding volumes, numbers 2 to 4, spanned the break in the calendar year.

Reportedly 500 copies of each part were published and "A limited number of the Report is for sale, and may be had by addressing the University Press,

Liverpool. Price 10/6 per annum". A review of the second part of Volume 3 appearing in the British Medical Journal gave the price as 5s 6d (*BMJ* 1901;2:717). Whether there were subscribers, or how the journal was funded, was not stated.

A change of the journal's name occurred with the fifth volume, published in 1903, to the even more unwieldy *Thompson Yates and Johnston Laboratories Report*. A brief Preface to this "New Series" explained the name change:

> The munificent gift of Mr. William Johnston has placed beside the existing Thompson Yates Laboratories a laboratory for Bio-Chemistry, Tropical Medicine, Experimental Medicine, and Comparative Pathology. These laboratories are occupied and directed by workers who have already collaborated in the Thompson Yates Report. It has, therefore, seemed as natural as it is desirable to now issue the work emanating from the two sets of laboratories in a single publication. The present volume is the first of a new series that we hope may continue to flow from the Thompson Yates and Johnston Laboratories in conjunction, evidencing the utility and fruitfulness of the generous gift with which the public-spirited founders have equipped the University of their city. [capitals in original].

Unlike the "old series", page numbering was not consecutive for first and second parts in volumes 5 and 6. Only a single part appeared in volume 7. No statement was included as to why the Journal ended at this point; perhaps insufficient material was available, or perhaps authors understandably wanted their publications to be available to a broader readership than that accessing a laboratory house journal.

Commentary

The *Thompson Yates Laboratories Report* and the *Thompson Yates and Johnston Laboratories Report* may be little known, likewise Sherrington's role in their editing. The journal is not mentioned per se in Liddell's (1952) obituary notice of Sherrington, although the bibliography (prepared by John Fulton) does list six publications therein by Sherrington, likewise in Denny-Brown's (1939) compilation. One might increase this to seven if the Addendum to Grünbaum & Sherrington's (1901–1902) paper is counted as a separate publication (all are listed in the References section below, and the citations may differ in places from those appearing in Liddell). These works by Sherrington appear in the first, fourth, and fifth volumes and most were reprinted from elsewhere rather than presenting new information. Others associated with Sherrington who also published in the Journal were Robert S. Woodworth and William B. Warrington.

A cursory examination of the journal contents suggests that, after the first volume, papers related to physiology were very much in the minority, so from an editorial perspective the workload for Sherrington may have been minimal. Papers related to bacteriology and to tropical medicine prevailed, and I would doubt that Sherrington took great interest in these, perhaps deferring to his co-editor Boyce for decisions on their publication. There were no editorials, but two "In Memoriam" pieces were credited to the joint editors.

All issues of the *Thompson Yates Laboratories Report* and the *Thompson Yates and Johnston Laboratories Report* are accessible via Internet Archive, and hard copies may be viewed at the Special Collections and Archives at the University of Liverpool (Sydney Jones Library).

Acknowledgements

Unpublished manuscript, 2024.

References

Denny-Brown D (ed.). *Selected writings of Sir Charles Sherrington. A testimonial presented by the neurologists forming the Guarantors of the journal Brain.* Oxford: Oxford University Press, 1939 [1979].

Liddell EGT. Charles Scott Sherrington 1857–1952. *Obit Not Fell R Soc* 1952; 8: 241–270.

Sherrington CS. On the spinal animal. (Marshall Hall lecture.) *Thomp Yates Lab Rep* 1898–1899; 1: 27–44.

Sherrington CS. Experiments in examination of the peripheral distribution of the fibres of the posterior roots of some spinal nerves. *Thomp Yates Lab Re* 1898–1899; 1: 45–173.

Sherrington CS. On the innervation of antagonistic muscles. Sixth note. *Thomp Yates Lab Rep* 1898–1899; 1: 175–176.

Grünbaum ASF, Sherrington CS. Observations on the physiology of the cerebral cortex of some of the higher apes. *Thomp Yates Lab Rep* 1901–1902; 4: 351–354.

Sherrington CS. Addendum on the pyramidal tracts. *Thomp Yates Lab Rep* 1901–1902; 4: 355.

Grünbaum ASF, Sherrington CS. Observations on the physiology of the cerebral cortex of the anthropoid apes. *Thomp Yates Lab Rep* 1903; 5: 55–58.

Sherrington CS, Sowton SCM. On the dosage of the mammalian heart by chloroform. *Thomp Yates Lab Rep* 1903; 5, 69–104.

Table: *Thompson Yates (and Johnston) Laboratories Report* contents by volume

NB The titles of some articles differ between the tables of Contents and the title page of the paper (the latter has been preferred).

Volume 1 (1898-1899): *Thompson Yates Laboratories Report*

Reference	Title	Author(s)
	Preface.	–
I: 1–18	Description of the laboratories.	–
I: 19–23	Social dreams. Being an address given to the medical students of University College Liverpool, by the Rev. S. A. Thompson Yates, M.A., on the opening of the session 1899–1900.	S. A. Thompson Yates
I: 27–44	On the spinal animal. Being the Marshall Hall Prize Address by Charles S. Sherrington, M.A., M.D., F.R.S.	Charles S. Sherrington
I: 45–173	Experiments in examination of the peripheral distribution of the fibres of the posterior roots of some spinal nerves.	Charles S. Sherrington
I: 175–176	On the innervation of antagonistic muscles. Sixth note.	Charles S. Sherrington
I: 177–195	Observations on the anatomy, physiology and degenerations of the nervous system of the bird.	Rubert Boyce and W.B. Warrington
I: 197–210	On the structural alterations observed in nerve cells.	W.B. Warrington
I: 211–221	Further observations on the structural alterations observed in nerve cells.	W.B. Warrington
I: 223–228	The morbid anatomy of a case of lead paralysis. Condition of the nerves, muscles, muscle spindles, and spinal cord.	E.E. Laslett and W.B. Warrington
I: 229–233	Observations on the ascending tracts in the spinal cord of the human subject.	E.E. Laslett and W.B. Warrington
I: 235–238	Note on muscle-spindles in pseudo-hypertrophic paralysis.	Albert S. Grünbaum

Volume 2 (1898–1899): *Thompson Yates Laboratories Report*

Reference	Title	Author(s)
II: 1–8	Blood and the identification of bacterial species.	Albert S. Grünbaum
II: 9–11	Note on the specific action of normal human serum upon the bacillus coli communis.	S. R. Christophers
II: 13–15	The bacteriological diagnosis of plague.	C. Balfour Stewart
II: 17	Preliminary note on some experiments to determine the comparative efficacy of the different constituents of Haffkine's plague prophylactic.	C. Balfour Stewar t
II: 19–22	Experiments to determine the efficacy of the different constituents of Haffkine's plague prophylactic.	C. Balfour Stewart
II: 23–25	A new micrococcus with a note on the bacteriology of lymphadenoma.	J. Hill Abram
II: 27–28	Mouse favus.	J. Hill Abram
II: 29–35	Tubercle bacilli in milk, butter, and margarine.	H.E. Annett
II: 37–40	A classification of the micro-organisms found in water.	R.W. Boyce and C.A. Hill
II: 41–44	Parliamentary powers for the sanitary supervision and control of ice-cream manufacture.	E. Petronell Manby
II: 45–52	Meat inspection and the abolition of private slaughterhouses.	E. Petronell Manby
II: 53–55	The disinfection of the excreta.	C.A. Hill and J. Hill Abram
II: 57–67	Boric acid and formalin as milk preservatives.	H.E. Annett
II: 69–71	Carcinoma of the kidney arising in the glomeruli.	J. Hill Abram
II: 73–77	Two cases of lympho-sarcoma with remarks upon the differential diagnosis of some general glandular enlargements.	J. Hill Abram
II: 79–89	The morbid anatomy and pathology of Dr. Bradshaw's case of myelopathic albumosuria.	Thos. R. Bradshaw and W.B. Warrington
II: 91–92	Report of the School of Physiology. Year 1899.	–
II: 93–96	Report of the School of Pathology.	–
II: 97–111	Report to the Medical Officer of Health of Liverpool of the samples analyzed during the year 1898.	–
II: 113–118	The bacteriological investigations undertaken for the Water Committee of the City of Liverpool.	–
II: 119–121	The Pathological Diagnosis Society of Liverpool.	W.B. Warrington
II: 123	Museum Report, 1899.	–
II: 125	Comparative pathology Report.	J.F. Ryder
II: 127	Report of the Holt Fellow in Pathology.	E.E. Glynn
II: 127	The Colonial Fellowship.	–
II: 127	Report of the Alexander Fellow.	A. Stanley Griffith

(continued)

Reference	Title	Author(s)
II: 129–133	Preliminary report on ophthalmia. Histological appearance of an acutely inflamed conjunctiva.	– [A. Stanley Griffith]
II: 135–143	The Liverpool School of Tropical Medicine Report for 1899.	A.H. Milne
II: 145–147	Library. Periodicals taken by departmental library.	–
Supplement (1–60)	Oysters and disease. An account of certain observations upon the normal and pathological histology of the oyster and other shellfish.	W.A. Herdamn and R. Boyce
Supplement (1–61)	Report of the malaria expedition of the Liverpool School of Tropical Medicine and Medical Parasitology.	R. Ross, H.E. Annett, E.E. Austen

Volume 3 (1900–1901): *Thompson Yates Laboratories Report*

Reference	Title	Author(s)
III: 1–29	The distribution of bacterium coli commune.	Harriette Chick
III: 31–38	On the distribution of bacillus enteritidis sporogenes.	C. Balfour Stewart
III: 39–40	Apparatus for heating cultures to separate spore-bearing micro-organisms.	C. Balfour Stewart
III: 40	Description of photographs of cultures of B. pestis in broth showing 'stalactite' formation.	Balfour Stewart
III: 41–57	Experiments on the differentiation and isolation from mixtures of the bacillus coli communis and bacillus typhosus by the use of sugars and the salts of bile.	Alfred MacConkey
III: 59–70	Note upon the action of the Dibdin contact beds constructed by the Corporation of Liverpool at West Derby.	–
III: 71–73	Note upon the two species of 'fungus' commonly found in sewage contaminated water.	R. Boyce
III: 75–78	Preservatives and colouring matters in food.	E.W. Hope
III: 79–99	Report to the Medical Officer of Health of the investigations and analyses made by the Corporation bacteriologist.	–
III: 101–108	The distribution of tuberculosis in Liverpool.	J.H. Elliott
III: 109–115	Note on experiments on sewage disposal in Germany.	A.S. Grünbaum
III: 117–129	The distribution of B. coli commune.	Harriette Chick
III: 131–150	The relation between bacillus enteritidis sporogenes of Klein and diarrhoea.	E.E. Klein

Reference	Title	Author(s)
III: 151–154	Further note on bile salt lactose agar.	Alfred MacConkey
III: 155–157	Note on the staining of flagella.	Alfred MacConkey
III: 159–164	Report on a primary malignant growth of the kidney.	Keith Monsarrat
III: 165–167	In Memoriam. [Walter Myers]	–
III: 169–176	The prevention of malaria in tropical Africa.	S.R. Christophers
III: 177–181	Enlarged spleens and malaria.	C.W. Daniels
III: 183–188	Diagrams illustrating the life-history of the parasites of malaria.	R. Ross and R. Fielding-Ould
III: 189–268	Report of the malaria expedition to Nigeria of the Liverpool School of Tropical Medicine and Medical Parasitology.	H.E. Annett, J. Everett Dutton, and J.H. Elliott

Volume 4 (1901–1902): *Thompson Yates Laboratories Report*

Reference	Title	Author(s)
IV: 1–92	Report of the malaria expedition to Nigeria of the Liverpool School of Tropical Medicine and Medical Parasitology. Part II. Filariasis.	H.E. Annett, J. Everett Dutton, and J.H. Elliott
IV: Appendix i-xxi Bibliography i-xiv	Notes on a collection of mosquitoes from West Africa and description of a new species.	F.V. Theobald
IV: 93–96	The hibernation of English mosquitoes.	H.E. Annett and J. Everett Dutton
IV: 99–148	The flora of the conjunctiva in health and disease.	A. Stanley Griffith
IV: 151–165	Bile salt broth.	Alfred MacConkey and Charles A. Hill
IV: 169–174	Milk as a vehicle of tubercle and present local legislation in regard to it.	E.W. Hope
IV: 177–179	The excretory and tubercular contamination of milk.	R. Boyce
IV: 183–199	Report to the Medical Officer of the bacteriological examinations made for the city of Liverpool during the year 1900.	R. Boyce
IV: 203–205	Note on 'pink-eye' in horses.	C. Balfour Stewart and R. Boyce
IV: 209–212	Report of the librarian.	A.S. Grünbaum
IV: 213–347	The injury current of nerve. The key to its physical structure.	J.S. Macdonald

(continued)

Reference	Title	Author(s)
IV: 351–354	Observations on the physiology of the cerebral cortex of some of the higher apes.	A.S.F. Grünbaum and C.S. Sherrington
IV: 355	Addendum on the pyramidal tracts.	C.S. Sherrington
IV: 359–368	Tubercular expectoration in public thoroughfares: an experimental inquiry.	H.E. Annet
IV: 371–376	Pseudo Actinomyces of the udder of the cow.	R. Boyce
IV: 379–382	An isolated case of plague.	A. Stanley Griffith
IV: 385–406	A new pathogenic bacillus isolated from a case diagnosed as typhoid fever with a summary of fourteen similar cases hitherto reported.	Edward H. Hume
IV: 409–414	Note upon fungus deposits in unfiltered water mains.	R. Boyce
IV: 417–429	Sulphide producing organisms.	E.N. Coutts
IV: 433–437	A new nitrometer for the clinical estimation of urea by the hypobromite process.	W.G. Little
IV: 441–446	Extensive focal necrosis of the liver in early typhoid fever.	E.E. Glynn
IV: 449–451	Multiple aneurisms of the aorta.	J. Hill Abram and Lyn Dimond
IV: 455–468	Preliminary note upon a trypanosome occurring in the blood of man.	J. Everett Dutton
IV: 471–474	Quelques notes sur les embryons de 'Strongyloides intestinalis' et leur pénétration par le peau.	Paul Van Durme
IV: 479–563	Report of the yellow fever expedition to Parà of the Liverpool School of Tropical Medicine and Medical Parasitology.	H.E. Durham

Volume 5 (1903): *Thompson Yates and Johnston Laboratories Report*

Reference	Title	Author(s)
	Preface.	–
V (Part 1): 1–11	The opening of the Johnston laboratories.	–
V (Part 1): 15–17	The national importance of the study of tropical veterinary medicine.	Professor Nocard
V (Part 1): 21–52	On the synthesis of fats accompanying absorption from the intestine, and on the limitations of synthesis by enzymes and by living cells, respectively.	Benjamin Moore
V (Part 1): 55–58	Observations on the physiology of the cerebral cortex of the anthropoid apes.	A.S.F. Grünbaum and C.S. Sherrington
V (Part 1): 61–66	The electrical conductivity of mammalian nerve.	R.S. Woodworth

Reference	Title	Author(s)
V (Part 1): 69–104	On the dosage of the mammalian heart by chloroform.	C.S. Sherrington and S.C.M. Sowton
V (Part 1): 107–113	Experiments on the detection of B. typhosus in infected material.	Edward H. Hume
V (Part 1): 117–118	The thick-film process for the detection of organisms in the blood.	Ronald Ross
V (Part 1): 121–122	Note on the staining of bacterial flagella with silver.	J.W.W. Stephens
V (Part 1): 125–129	A preliminary note on the supposed bactericidal influence of flour and allied substances on bacillus typhosus.	Herbert E. Roaf
V (Part 1): 133–163	The relation of vesicular mole to chorion carcinoma.	J. Effie Prowse
V (Part 1): 167–184	On a characteristic organism associated with cancer of the breast.	Keith W. Monsarrat
V (Part 1): 187–189	'Tick fever' in man.	Cuthbert Christie
V (Part 1): 193–218	Blackwater fever.	J.W.W. Stephens
V (Part 1): 221–233	Summary of researches on native malaria and malarial prophylaxis; on black-water fever: its nature and prophylaxis.	J.W.W. Stephens and S.R. Christophers
Supplement (1–46)	Report of the malaria expedition to the Gambia 1902 of the Liverpool School of Tropical Medicine and Medical Parasitology.	J. Everett Dutton
Appendix (i–xi)	Report on a collection of mosquitoes or Culicidae, etc., from Gambia, and descriptions of new species.	F.V. Theobald
	In Memoriam Rev. Samuel Ashton Thompson Yates, M.A.	C.S.S., R.B.
	In Memoriam Professor Nocard.	C.S.S., R.B.
V (Part 2): 1–57	First report of the trypanosomiasis expedition to Senegambia (1902) of the Liverpool School of Tropical Medicine and Medical Parasitology.	J. Everett Dutton and John L. Todd
Appendix (i–iii)	New Culicid from Senegal and notes on the species of mosquitoes, etc.	F.V. Theobald
V (Part 2): 79–82	A new parasite of man.	Ronald Ross
V (Part 2): 85–86	Note on the discovery of *Trypanosoma gambiense*, Dutton.	R. Ross and R.W. Boyce
V (Part 2): 89–101	Bacteria in public swimming baths.	Ernest Glynn and J.C. Matthews
V (Part 2): 105–107	Parasitic disease in the haddock (Gadus aeglefinus).	J.W.W. Stephens and Rubert Boyce

Volume 6 (1904): Thompson Yates and Johnston Laboratories Report

Reference	Title	Author(s)
VI (Part 1): 1–112	Reports of the trypanosomiasis expedition to the Congo 1903–1904 of the Liverpool School of Tropical Medicine and Medical Parasitology.	J. Everett Dutton, John L. Todd and Cuthbert Christy
VI (Part 1): 115–117	A new haemogregarine in an African toad.	J.W.W. Stephens
VI (Part 1): 119–121	Two cases on intestinal myiasis.	J.W.W. Stephens
VI (Part 1): 123–124	Note on the pathology of tropical 'swellings'.	J.W.W. Stephens
VI (Part 1): 125–126	Non-flagellate typhoid bacilli.	J.W.W. Stephens
VI (Part 1): 129–135	Cladorchis watsoni (Conygham). A human parasite from Africa.	A.E. Shipley
VI (Part 1): 139–147	The intermediary host of filaria cypseli.	J. Everett Dutton
VI (Part 1): 151–191	An experimental study of the physical chemistry of anaesthesia in relationship to its causation.	Benjamin Moore and Herbert E. Roaf
VI (Part 1): 195–198	On the action of chloroform on the proteids of serum and upon solutions of haemoglobin.	E.S. Edie
VI (Part 1): 201–205	A simple method for the preparation and determination of lecithin.	Herbert E. Roaf and E.S. Edie
VI (Part 2): 1–95	Report on trypanosomes, trypanosomiasis, and sleeping sickness being an experimental investigation into their pathology and treatment.	H. Wolferstan Thomas
VI (Part 2): 97–102	Gland puncture in trypanosomiasis compared with other methods of demonstrating the presence of the parasite. Fourth interim report. From the expedition of the Liverpool School of Tropical Medicine to the Congo 1903.	The late J. Everett Dutton and John L. Todd
VI (Part 2): 111–128	The nature of human tick-fever in the Eastern part of the Congo free state with notes on the distribution and bionomics of the tick.	The late J. Everett Dutton and John L. Todd
VI (Part 2): 131–136	On the external anatomy of Ornithodoros moubata (Murray).	Robert Newstead
VI (Part 2): 139–141	On the habits of the marine mosquito (Acartomyia Zammith, Theobald).	E.H. Ross

Volume 7 (1905): Thompson Yates and Johnston Laboratories Report

Reference	Title	Author(s)
VII: 3–6	On a new pathogenic louse which acts as the intermediary host of a new haemogregarine in the blood of the Indian field rat (Jerbellus indicus).	S.R. Christophers and R. Newstead
VII: 9–12	Note on the anatomy of Gastrodiscus hominis (Lewis and McConnell, 1876).	J.W.W. Stephens
VII: 15–72	A revison of the Sarcopsyllidae: a family of Siphonaptera.	Karl Jordan and The Hon. N. Charles Rothschild
VII: 75–88	The maiotic process in mammalia.	J.E.S. Moore and C.E. Walker

Book reviews

1. Philosophical foundations of neuroscience (2nd edition)

[Bennett MR, Hacker PMS. Wiley Blackwell, 2022]

The first edition of this book appeared in 2003, when I happened to be the book review editor for *Advances in Clinical Neuroscience and Rehabilitation* (*ACNR*). Sadly, no review copy was received and hence no review appeared, so it would now seem time, with the kind permission of the current *ACNR* book review editor, to make amends. This requires a brief summary of some key aspects of the first edition (452 pages of text!) as well as the new additions, amounting to around 70000 words, in the second (525 pages of text!).

The book argues for the importance of conceptual analysis, informed by the logico-grammatical approach to philosophy developed by (amongst others) Wittgenstein, in the interpretation of the empirical findings of neuroscience research, particularly in the domain of cognitive neuroscience. One of the key contentions is that neuroscientists have applied to the brain concepts which logically can apply only to the human being, a shortcoming which Max Bennett (a neuroscientist) and Peter Hacker (a philosopher) term the "mereo-logical fallacy in neuroscience", mereology being the logic of part/whole relations. Pervasive ideas in neuroscience are characterised as conceptually incoherent, for example the notion that what one remembers, the ability to recollect, is dependent upon something stored or encoded in the brain (surely a commonplace belief amongst cognitive neurologists). To be sure, a function-ing brain is required for the exercise of these (and other) powers, capacities, or faculties, and structural and functional changes within the brain may under-pin their development and persistence, but conceptually the brain does not store or encode anything.

As well as the methodological chapters, the various domains of neuro-science are systematically examined: sensation, perception, cognition, conation, volition, emotion, consciousness and self-consciousness. The argu-ments are presented within the historical context of the development of neuroscientific ideas from Aristotle to the present (expanded on elsewhere[1]) with direct citations from the works of many neuroscientists, both historical (e.g. Sherrington, Eccles) and contemporary (e.g. Edelman, Blakemore, Sperry, Weiskrantz) used to illustrate the misconceptions, entanglements, or confusions which Bennett and Hacker detect. For example, the new edition takes on Tononi's Integrated Information Theory and Dehaene's Global Workspace Theory, and both are found conceptually wanting. At least one error remains from the first edition: Thomas Willis is described (p.38) as the

"Professor of Medicine at Oxford" rather than the Sedleian Professor of Natural Philosophy (a curious error for the Oxonian Hacker to make).

The authors' aim was to produce a handbook which could assist neuroscientists in their conceptual approach to the issues they study, but not to question their empirical findings. However, many neuroscientists didn't like this intervention, however helpfully intended, and many philosophers hated it, particularly those (e.g. Dennett, Searle) whose ideas were rebutted, prompting a further volume to air these disagreements.[2] I suspect that many, probably most, neurologists will not find this a straightforward read and indeed may not persist in reading from cover to cover. Even for those of a philosophical persuasion it is a tough (but necessary, salutary) read, in part because of the unfamiliar idiom – despite the co-authorship, this is evidently largely the work of Hacker rather than Bennett. Some readers will undoubtedly reject the arguments, others may be intrigued by them, others may adopt the conceptual approach. Although the relation to empirical neuroscience research is explored in greater depth in the companion volume,[1] the possibilities of the conceptual approach to clinical neurology have yet to be explored in any depth.

Acknowledgements

Unpublished manuscript, mid-2022.

References

1. Bennett MR, Hacker PMS. *History of cognitive neuroscience.* Chichester: Wiley-Blackwell, 2008.
2. Bennett M, Dennett D, Hacker P, Searle J. *Neuroscience and philosophy. Brain, mind, and language.* New York: Columbia University Press, 2007.

2. Victor Horsley. The world's first neurosurgeon and his conscience

[Aminoff MJ. Cambridge University Press, 2022]

Michael Aminoff will be well known to many neurologists for his edited textbook *Neurology in General Medicine* (now eponymous, *Aminoff's*, in its 6th edition, published 2021) and by historians of neurology for his work on Brown-Séquard. Now he turns his attention to another giant in the history of the development of the clinical and experimental neurosciences, Victor Horsley (1857–1916). Evidently, however, the idea for this biography is (very) long-standing: the author interviewed Francis Walshe (1885–1973), formerly Horsley's house surgeon, in 1966, but deferred writing after another biography of Horsley appeared in that year.

The book documents Horsley's prodigious skills, as both an experimenter and as a clinician, facilitated by being in the right places at the right time and knowing many influential figures in the growing disciplines of neuroscience in the late 19th and early 20th centuries. In his late twenties he became professor-superintendent of the Brown Institution in London, pursuing studies of the thyroid gland and rabies (he was succeeded in this post by Sherrington). Thereafter he worked on cortical localization studies in animals, following the experimental lead of Ferrier and the theoretical lead of Hughlings Jackson, developing skills which were crucial to his subsequent success as one of the first neurosurgeons, working at the National Hospital, Queen Square. He is also remembered for developing the first stereotactic apparatus (along with RH Clarke).

As if these clinical achievements were not enough, Horsley also had energy for medical politics (MDU, GMC, BMA) and other causes (temperance, women's suffrage) and seemed to relish conflict with those persuaded of ideas contrary to his own (e.g. the antivivisectionists). In his late 50s he joined the war effort and deployed his extensive organizational skills in trying to improve medical services, an effort which ultimately resulted in his untimely death from "heatstroke" in Mesopotamia in 1916.

The name of Horsley may be familiar to many practitioners of the neuro-disciplines, perhaps neurosurgeons more so than neurologists, but probably deserves to be better known. Here at the Walton Centre in Liverpool there is a ward named for him, the Horsley ITU (we also have a ward named for Sherrington) but I wonder how many of those working there know anything of the man. We should be thankful to Dr Aminoff for returning, after many decades, to his plan for this biography. The result is an engaging read, well-illustrated, which has delved into the many facets of Horsley's life, both clinical and non-clinical.

As it happens, I reviewed Aminoff's first biography, *Brown-Séquard: A Visionary of Science*, many years ago (in *Cambridge Medicine (Journal of the University of Cambridge Clinical School)* 1994;**11(1)**:48), and the opportunity to read this further example of the author's skills as a biographer has afforded similar edification and enjoyment.

Acknowledgements

Unpublished manuscript, end 2022.

3. The idea of epilepsy. A medical and social history of epilepsy in the modern era (1860–2020)

[Simon Shorvon. Cambridge University Press, 2023]

Anyone interested in the history of epilepsy will find themselves, sooner or later, consulting Owsei Temkin's *The falling sickness. A history of epilepsy from the Greeks to the beginnings of modern neurology*. First published in 1945 and fully revised in 1971, the book was informed by Temkin's (1902–2002) deep historical and linguistic scholarship, including quotations from Latin, ancient Greek, Italian, French, German, and even Arabic sources. However, as his title indicated, Temkin chose not to pursue his study beyond the beginnings of modern neurology which he placed, not unreasonably, in the "age of Hughlings Jackson", hence effectively the 1860s to 1890s. Students of the history of epilepsy who consult Temkin are thus inevitably left with the question: what happened next?

Step forward Simon Shorvon to take up the gauntlet. With something approaching fifty years of clinical experience in the epilepsy field, a prolific author with a fluid prose style, and also acknowledged for some significant contributions to the history of neurology (e.g. the International League Against Epilepsy; and the National Hospital, Queen Square, London, co-authored with Alistair Compston), one can think of no one better suited to take on this daunting task.

He uses the metaphor of voyage to inform his approach, the core of the book comprising five long chronological chunks covering 1860 and 2020, the last three encompassing 25–year periods from the end of the second world war onwards. Whilst the temptation might have been to focus on specific individuals and researches in the clinical arena (a "Whiggish" history"), Professor Shorvon has wisely broadened his horizons to take in societal responses to epilepsy and persons with epilepsy, and also the experience of having epilepsy as documented in literary works and film, thereby providing a much richer coverage than found in Temkin (although he did conclude with a section on "The world of the epileptic" which, inter alia, discussed some of the works of Dostoyevsky).

As might be expected, the book is particularly good on Queen Square contributions (Hughlings Jackson, Victor Horsley) and on the institutional history of international epilepsy organisations and their meetings and debates. From the medical perspective, there is excellent coverage of therapeutic, surgical, neuroimaging and genetic advances in epilepsy. The ghastly history of eugenics as applied to persons with epilepsy is covered in detail. The book is illustrated with original, and arresting, artwork by David Cobley.

To select one or two examples which fall within my particular spheres of interest, there is welcome discussion of the epilepsy colony movement which, beginning in the late 19th century, segregated epileptics from society in (generally) rural settings where they worked and were cared for. Although retrospectively we may consider the colony function to be nothing more than custodial, it may be that contemporaneously these were enlightened and beneficial havens for persons with epilepsy compared with general society. Incidentally, I'm not persuaded (p.100) that the Chalfont Centre for Epilepsy predated the Maghull Home in Liverpool by 4 years (1884 vs 1888), an assertion which sounds like special pleading from someone professionally associated with the former and runs contrary to the evidence of which I am aware. As for literary depictions of epilepsy, it is good to find several pages (pp.381–6) devoted to the work of the author Margiad Evans (1909–1958) whose *A Ray of Darkness* (1952) was one of the first patient accounts of epilepsy (both author and book are given incorrectly at p.547).

Many other typographical errors, some jarring, occur, e.g. would any author knowingly say of their work that part thereof is "dealt with less comprehensibly" (p.14), rather than "less comprehensively"? Other egregious examples: Henry VIII bans university study of physiognomy in 1551 (p.42n40), i.e. four years after his death (1547); Paul Broca's finding of cerebral localisation of speech expression is given as 1871 (p.74) rather than 1861; and Richard Caton's demonstration of the intrinsic electrical currents of the brain is dated 1885 (p.211) rather than 1875.

These quibbles aside, overall this book is a terrific read, indeed required reading, I would suggest, for anyone with an interest in epilepsy per se, not just its history.

Acknowledgements

Unpublished manuscript, 2023.

4. Thomas Willis 1621 – 1675: his life and work

[J. Trevor Hughes. Royal Society of Medicine, 1991]

Thomas Willis was the most distinguished physician of his day and a natural philosopher of international renown, a status achieved principally as a result of his experimental researches performed in Oxford in the 1660s. Trevor Hughes has coupled a distinguished career in neuropathology in Oxford with a long-standing interest in Willis (who may be described as the first Oxford neuropathologist); the latter studies are brought to a culmination with this short book (151 pages) on Willis's life and work, published by the Royal Society of Medicine in the Eponymists in Medicine series.

In setting out the little that is known of Willis's early life (chapters 1 to 6), the author provides an account of the historical milieu in which Willis grew up. His education at Christ Church, Oxford, coincided with the English Civil War and the upheavals in the University enforced by the Parliamentary Visitors after the defeat of the King. As a staunch Royalist, Willis was out of favour until the restoration of the monarchy in 1660, shortly after which he was appointed to the Sedleian Chair of Natural Philosophy. This prompted Willis's study of the brain which resulted in the publication in 1664 of his most famous work, generally known as *Cerebri anatome*.

Experimental philosophy flourished in the third quarter of the 17th century in Oxford, a period which has been enlighteningly documented by Robert G. Frank in his book *Harvey and the Oxford physiologists. A study of scientific ideas* (Berkeley: University of California Press, 1980), a work to which Hughes acknowledges his debt and from which he quotes several pages verbatim at one point. Brief sketches of the significant scientific figures of the day who were most influential on Willis and his studies are given, including Robert Boyle, Christopher Wren, and Richard Lower, the anatomist who performed many of the dissections for *Cerebri anatome*.

Probably the strongest section of the book is that devoted to Willis's scientific and medical publications and the assessment of his contributions to neuroanatomy and clinical medicine. These chapters (7 to 10) include illustrations and quotations from the original works, including Wren's illustration from *Cerebri anatome* of the base of the brain showing the arterial circle upon which Willis's eponymous fame rests, although, as Hughes points out, he was far from being he first to describe or illustrate the anastomosis but the first to appreciate its physiological significance. Less well remembered although no less fascinating are Willis's clinical descriptions, including probably the first accounts of myasthenia gravis and restless legs syndrome.

The final chapters record Willis's move to London, where he became the most sought after physician of the day, his family, and his death. Past and present assessments of Willis and his work are included, but here there is a curious omission, namely the question of whether Willis misappropriated the work of his junior assistant, Richard Lower, and published it as his own in *Cerebri anatome*. Although alluded to in passing (p.111), there is no reference to the statements of Michael Foster in his influential *Lectures on the History of Physiology in the Sixteenth, Seventeenth, and Eighteenth Centuries* (Cambridge: Cambridge University Press, 1901) regarding the matter. Though Willis is probably absolved of any scientific misbehaviour, it would have been interesting to have read a full discussion of the case both for and against.

Although this book is far from being a definitive work of scholarship, there is much to interest and stimulate the reader, particularly those wanting an introduction to Willis and his work. The quality of the illustrations is excellent throughout. Unfortunately, the prose is not so elegant, Hughes having a tendency to repeat himself which I found increasingly irksome (for instance, a complete paragraph is reproduced almost verbatim on pages 101 and 107); this is compounded by numerous errors of spelling, dates, and cross-referencing which one would have expected to be corrected at the proof-reading stage. These criticisms aside, this is a book worth reading and, I would suggest, mandatory for Oxford medical students and budding neurologists.

Acknowledgements

Adapted from: Larner AJ. *Oxford Medical School Gazette* 1993;43(2):53.

5. The spice of life: from Northumberland to world neurology

[**Lord Walton of Detchant. Royal Society of Medicine, 1993**]

Lord Walton of Detchant is one of the most noted British neurologists of the post-World War 2 period. He is perhaps best known to medical students for his book *Essentials of Neurology*, now in its sixth edition, and to neurologists (in training or trained) for his revisions of *Brain's Diseases of the Nervous System*. He was instrumental in the development of a neurology department of national and international renown at Newcastle-upon-Tyne in the 1960s and 1970s ("Neurocastle"), eventually becoming Dean of the Medical School. He has also achieved the distinction of being, at various times, president of the British Medical Association, the Royal Society of Medicine, the Association of British Neurologists, the General Medical Council, and the World Federation of Neurology. For these services he was raised to the peerage in 1989. Clearly his has been a full life with much to relate, and one is therefore not surprised by the length of this book (643 pages), written, so the Preface tells us, at the suggestion of family members and friends.

However, from the vantage point of a neurologist in training, the content is disappointing. Although he alludes to his interests in muscle disease, particularly muscular dystrophy and inflammatory muscle disease, there is no significant account of his research work, only of those researchers with whom he collaborated. Furthermore, clinical anecdotes, the grist of a good medical (auto)biography, occur but infrequently. Rather, we are regaled with the minutiae of Lord Walton's personal activities, including chapters on his sporting interests (including an unpalatable section on "golf courses I have known"), the Territorial Army, and a year-by-year account of his international travel to attend conferences and give lectures. For one not acquainted with the author, this is dreary stuff indeed, and the long section of reminiscences of his work on various committees does nothing to lighten the tone. He mentions at one point, not without a hint of pride, that he was once serving concurrently on 146 local, national, and international committees! Needless to say, such demands necessitated abandoning the practice of clinical neurology. There are frequent vignettes of colleagues (invariably "distinguished" and/or "outstanding") and he recalls many dinners attended in the course of his work (frequently "oenological" and occasionally "Rabelaisian").

The Preface tells us that the book was initially intended for private circulation amongst family and friends, and this is the audience who will enjoy it most. Perhaps a very different book would have emerged if the general public or the neurological community had been its principal target readership. Despite the mass of detail, I was left with little insight into the man, or his neurological achievements.

Acknowledgements

Unpublished manuscript, ca. 1993–4.

6. Queen Square. A history of the National Hospital and its Institute of Neurology

[S Shorvon, A Compston. Cambridge University Press, 2019]

There can be few neurologists, if any, unaware of the signification of "Queen Square" (although in Liverpool it is synonymous with a bus station!). It used to be said that there were only two types of Neurologist – those who trained at Queen Square, and those who wished they had trained at Queen Square. Certainly many of the former and quite possibly many of the latter may be interested to consult this long awaited and limited edition history of an institution which some may still regard as the Neurology "mother ship".

The founding of the National Hospital in 1860 occurred at a time of developing interest in Neurology as an independent specialty (e.g. the work of Charcot and Vulpian at the Salpêtrière in Paris; Silas Weir Mitchell at the Turner's Lane Hospital in Philadelphia). Its origins were as a philanthropic endeavour funded by charity with unpaid honorary clinical appointments, from which has eventually evolved a research-intensive medical specialism. The journey documented here has evidently been a bumpy ride, with the hospital near closure on more than one occasion. Whilst the clinical contributions emanating from Queen Square are well known, the bureaucratic history provided here is certainly less familiar, and serves to remind us that the power struggle between clinicians and managers is not unique to our own times.

Great though the pantheon of QS alumni is, this book is no mere exercise in hagiography: although the greats are individually attended to (e.g. Hughlings Jackson, Ferrier, Gowers, Horsley, Holmes, Kinnier Wilson, Critchley, Symonds), this is also a carefully contextualised history, with much recourse to the minutes of the Board of Management and reference to contemporary historical events (hence, it is more than might have been anticipated from the book's title alone). The world wars in particular did much to shape the institution's history. The chapter on development of Neurology in the United Kingdom more widely is a welcome counterpoint; of course, Queen Square trainees accounted for much of the initial spread of neurological services.

This is a fascinating history, well told, with a uniformity of style despite the dual authorship and the (unspecified) contributions of three others (Andrew Lees, Michael Clark, Martin Rossor). The text is supplemented with footnotes, some quite extensive (e.g. biographical sketches of some of the notable, but not stellar, QS staff), black and white illustrations (some very evocative, such as the entrance hall where one sat before interview took place in the Boardroom, p.41; the blackboards in the lecture theatre, p.135; A-room, p.458–9). There are occasional anecdotes, consistently engaging (e.g. Carmichael's self-experimentation on testicular pain, p.441n4, was particularly eye-watering – researchers were made of stern stuff in those days!) and authorial asides.

It would be neglecting a reviewer's duty to forego a few minor criticisms, however nit-picking they may appear. There are occasional typographical and factual errors (particularly egregious: "Single Proton [*sic*] Emission Computed Tomography, p.399; the date given for Anita Harding's graduation, 1995, is in fact the year she died, p.474; "winter of discontent" ascribed to 1973/4, rather than 1978/9, p.503n14); many seem to be in the footnotes. I was disappointed that in discussing Gowers as a possible source for Arthur Conan Doyle's Sherlock Holmes story *The Resident Patient*, the reference (p.58n16) was to Lees' paper (*Brain* 2015;138:2103–8) but without mention of what I believe to be the original formulation of Holmes as Gowers (*The Sherlock Holmes Journal* 1992;20(4):128–30; Lees does not cite this paper, either) by Robin Howard and Hugh Willison, both of whom were working at QS at the time of publication. The minutiae of ward life and the patient perspective are also absent, since unlikely to have been recorded for the benefit of posterity.

I found this book an immensely enjoyable read. The authors have produced a work which will stand as the definitive history for many decades. They deserve our thanks and congratulations for their labours. It is a book which I shall certainly return to in the future.

Acknowledgements

Adapted from: Larner AJ. *Queen Square. A history of the National Hospital and its Institute of Neurology* by S Shorvon and A Compston. *Adv Clin Neurosci Rehabil* 2019;18(3):19.

7. Georges Gilles de la Tourette. Beyond the eponym

[O Walusinski. Oxford University Press, 2019]

Perhaps because of its euphony, the name of Georges Gilles de la Tourette often becomes embedded in the neurological consciousness at an early stage of clinical training, the more so from the association of his syndrome of motor and phonic tics with coprolalia, scatology being particularly memorable for some reason. But who knows anything about the man, other than perhaps his association with Charcot and the Salpêtrière school?

Olivier Walusinski has a long-established interest in the history of neurology in 19th century France (as well as of yawning), manifest in many journal publications. In this volume he shares his research into the life of GGdelaT, and it is a fascinating story: for example, how many neurologists can claim to have survived attempted assassination (in 1893)? For those with an interest in etymology, there is a helpful explanation of why the amputation to "Tourette" syndrome is incorrect, since based on a toponymic; if abbreviation is required, "Gilles" syndrome would be more appropriate.

By far the longest chapter in the book is, appropriately, devoted to the eponymous syndrome. I was always perplexed that the original report of 1884 (previously translated by Lajonchere et al., Arch Neurol 1996;53:567–74) was ostensibly devoted to startle syndromes ("jumping" of Maine, latah of Malaysia, and myriachit of Siberia) but it transpires that the tic disorder was then conceived to be related to these other disorders of excessive movement.

In addition, Walusinski gives a contextualised analysis of many of the other major publications, including a treatise on hysteria. Clearly Gilles de la Tourette was an indefatigable writer, also interested in biography (he wrote a work on the pioneer French journalist Renaudot). He himself had extensive interactions with journalists, not least to promote his own career, and wrote occasionally for the lay press under the nom de plume of Paracelsus. To what extent developing neurosyphilis may have contributed to some of his self-promoting actions ("megalomania") remains speculative.

Anyone interested in the origins of clinical neurology in late 19th century France will want to read this scholarly volume, which is well presented with many illustrations from the author's personal collection. There are a few niggly errors (e.g. "Helmotz", p.186, is presumably Helmholtz, as they share the same dates; Lucerne, p.112, should perhaps be Lausanne; figures numbers are inconsistent with those in the text in Chapter 8).

Acknowledgements

Adapted from: Larner AJ. *Georges Gilles de la Tourette. Beyond the eponym* by O Walusinski. *Adv Clin Neurosci Rehabil* 2019;18(4):29.

8. Sacred lives. An account of the history, cultural associations and social impact of epilepsy

[I Bone. Amazon, 2020. The Book Guild, 2022]

A recent ABN Newsletter drew my attention to this book by Ian Bone, a long serving (now retired) Consultant Neurologist in Glasgow. Prompted by the experience of caring for a son with epilepsy, this book has been written as an awareness raiser for a general audience, hence it is lightly rather than exhaustively referenced, although there is much here for Neurologists to learn from.

Whereas standard epilepsy texts focus on diagnosis, classification, investigation, and treatment (all briefly touched upon here), this book has more to say about epilepsy in the arts, the media, and society, as well as including a personal account of living with epilepsy. The book thus may be said to complement standard neurology texts, seamlessly bridging the gap between expert text and patient narrative. Only a brief flavour of the rich resulting melange can be given here.

With the benefit of the author's personal perspective, the sections on stigma and social isolation are particularly informative. Some of the history of this ostracism is also given, for example relating to the eugenics movement and the "epilepsy colony" movement, both originating in the nineteenth century. The author's clinical experience is to the fore in discussing legal ramifications of epilepsy. The legal subdivision of automatisms into sane and insane is indicative of the gulf that may exist between medical and legal thinking (p.263).

The many examples of the portrayal of individuals with epilepsy in books bespeaks an immense amount of reading. In addition, examples are also given from film, television, and other of the arts, resulting in a broad frame of cultural reference ranging from Dostoevsky to East Enders! The many inaccuracies in such portrayals are highlighted. Amongst the historical figures alleged to have had epilepsy who are discussed, I would have been intrigued to hear Dr. Bone's thoughts on the claim that St. Paul suffered from epilepsy.

Proceeds from the book will go to the William Quarrier Scottish Epilepsy Centre, in light of which I hope it will not seem churlish or mean-spirited to voice some minor criticisms. For example, it is not the case (p.29) that Chalfont St Peter was the first colony for people with epilepsy in the UK ("first patient admitted 1894"), since it was predated by the Maghull Home for Epileptics on the outskirts of Liverpool (first patient admitted 1888). Indeed, Maghull founding clinician, William Alexander (p.30), was asked for advice by the directors of the Chalfont colony, both at its foundation and some years later.

I'm also in disagreement with Ian Bone in his analysis of Shakespeare's *Othello*, where he seems ready to follow convention in diagnosing Othello with epilepsy (p.66–67), but all the eye-witness evidence is from Iago, hardly a reliable informant. I'm also sceptical that Dickens's character Walter Wilding, from the play *No Thoroughfare* (1867), has epilepsy (p.77).

There are a few typographical errors, the most egregious of which is "San Michael" for "San Michele" in the title of Axel Munthe's celebrated autobiography (p.171; an autocorrect? [NB corrected in The Book Guild edition, 2022]). The index is commendably thorough, a cut above the perfunctory apparatus one encounters in most textbooks these days.

There is a wealth of information in this book, evidently a labour of love. I highly recommend it to anyone involved in or interested in the care of people with epilepsy. At just £12 [NB Amazon edition, 2020], it's a steal!

Acknowledgements

Adapted from: Larner AJ. *Sacred lives. An account of the history, cultural associations and social impact of epilepsy* by I Bone. *Adv Clin Neurosci Rehabil* 2021;20(2):26.

Envoi: some thoughts on retirement from clinical medicine

… the spoken word is worth more than the written – if a choice can be made between things of no value.[1]

Essais. Michel de Montaigne. I:10 (On a ready or hesitant delivery)

If I were to present each of you with a binary forced-choice paradigm requiring you to decide whether I am a man of the spoken word or a man of the written word, I think many of you would choose the written word – and I would agree. I am more author than orator, being both bradyphrenic and inarticulate. But as today is about the spoken word, I shall rely on the written word to ensure that I don't omit anything that I want to say.

As you will know, Montaigne (1533–1592) took the decision in the early 1570s, when in his late 30s, to retire from his public life. [I digress here momentarily to note that the ancient Greeks had a specific word for a man who was merely a private citizen, as opposed to someone with a political office: *idiotes*. This word did not carry the pejorative connotations of our derivative word, idiot, to which I shall return at the end.] Montaigne returned to his chateau, located 40km east of Bordeaux, to his tower, in order to write his *Essais*. La tour comprised three levels: a chapel, a bedroom, and on the top floor his library, with quotations from his favourite classical authors written on the beams. I would like to tell you that I am retiring to my own personal library in the south of France – but unfortunately that is not true, just as it is not true that Montaigne retired from public life in the 1570s: he was twice mayor of Bordeaux in the 1580s before casting himself entirely as auteur in the late 1580s. Things are not always what they seem, although it is true that I shall be visiting (haunting?) libraries, like this one at the Liverpool Medical Institution.

So:

> All in vain, I will cease now
> My long absorption with the plough,
> With the tame and the wild creatures
> And man united with the earth.
> I have failed after many seasons
> To bring truth to birth,
> And nature's simple equations
> In the mind's precincts do not apply.

The opening verse of the poem *No through road*, the final work in the collection *Song at the year's turning*, published in 1955, by the Anglo-Welsh poet R.S. Thomas (1913–2000). I first encountered the work of RS around the age of 13; he was on the school English syllabus at that time. So what was it that attracted a shy, disaffected, alienated, adolescent schoolboy to these poems? And has caused him to return again and again to these works for almost 50 years? I think it is RS's sense of incompleteness, of falling short, of unfulfillment. In a word, his nihilism. If I adhere to any "ism" I think it is this one, although I would argue that it adheres to me, rather than the other way round. In which case, the more appropriate verb may be "inheres": this outlook, this valence, is inherent to my subjectivity, in the same way as, for example, colour blindness, or synaesthesia, or aphantasia is inherent to others – accepted as "the way things are", until other subjectivities are reported to be different.

But nihilism is not apathy, it is not a prospectus for inertia, it demands an active rather than a passive response. So, in that spirit, I wish to share with you briefly some of the secrets of my failure. Is an individual responsible for their own success or failure? Are success and failure legitimate categories of analysis? I think the notionally successful are as likely to claim yes, as the notionally failed are to say no. But I would suggest that if there are secrets of success and failure they are essentially the same, comprising: luck, fortune, chance, and contingency.

So, I was lucky:

- to be born in this country, at least at the time I was. The postwar consensus still held, there was still educational opportunity, and the potential for social mobility.
- to be born in Cirencester, a small town in south Gloucestershire, the capital of the Cotswolds; a town steeped in history, dating to its foundation in AD75 as the Roman Corinium Dobunnorum.
- to be born to fine parents, of working class origin, mother urban, father rural, whose formative years were shaped by the War. Accordingly, I think it is fair to say that they had no ambitions beyond those of making a home, raising a family, and enjoying the company of their extended families.
- to have an elder sister who could guide and advise me; some might say she sometimes bossed her little brother around, but not me!
- to be able to go to school, to learn, to be taught all kinds of fascinating things. [To her credit, I think my mother realised quite early that I was a "brainy" kid and might end up going to university, no doubt a source of great anxiety to her at a time when university students were generally perceived as kids with long hair who went on protest marches.]

But in addition to this pervasive, circumambient atmosphere of good fortune, something more is required, for which I use the term "liminal events". Liminality analysis embodies the idea of a threshold, inherent in the word liminal, from the Latin *limen*, indicating the possibility of change or transformation to a new state of being, applicable to both spatial and intellectual transitions. I first leaned about liminality from the late, great Dr Humphrey Fisher (1933–2019), who used the concept in his work as an African historian although it originated in cultural anthropology. As far as I am aware, such liminal transitions have no specified duration, indeed are of undetermined duration, so might encompass years, months, days, or might even be momentary (perhaps familiar as the "sliding doors" phenomenon).

So, for example, one morning in the lower sixth form, autumn 1980, walking into school across the playing field, as normal, I notice that the headmaster is out and about, bollocking kids who were smoking in the bike sheds. He sees me and asks, "So, Andrew, where are you going to university?". "I'm going to Leeds, sir." My recollection is that, at that time, there was a slim book listing all the university courses available in the UK, along with the A level grades required for entry, published by UCCA (later to become UCAS). I had looked up medicine, and found that entry to Leeds required three B grades, which I thought I could probably achieve.

I should say at this point that I have no recall of making a conscious, overt decision to study medicine, there was no epiphany, and certainly no vocation. (History of course now shows us that I had no aptitude for the subject, and certainly brought to it much ineptitude, indeed gross ineptitude.) I do recollect that one of our geography teachers, who doubled up as a part time "careers master", once said to me "Well, Andrew, you're going to pass all your exams, go to university, and be a doctor", and I had no better counter plan. Certainly I had spent some time in my formative years visiting hospitals following my father's accident, initially in 1974 when, after being knocked off his bike, he had a below knee amputation (perhaps the first neurological diagnosis I ever learned of was phantom limb pain). He also sustained an upper arm fracture which had pranged his radial nerve causing a wrist drop, so in 1976 he underwent elective surgery to arthrodese his wrist in a neutral position to give some function to his hand. I attended the hospital, Princess Margaret Hospital in Swindon (no longer in existence), with my parents some time later, where I recall that we sat around for a long time in a room with many other people, and a door would occasionally open and a name was called out: though I did not know it at the time, this was my first experience of an outpatient clinic! I think it was on that occasion that my father required an X-ray, whilst waiting for which I came across a small book, probably a nursing book, on anatomy and physiology, and thinking that looked very interesting!

Back to the headmaster, who was unimpressed with my Leeds plan. "Have you thought about Cambridge?". Well, yes, but only to conclude that it wasn't the kind of place for me: you apparently had to sit another exam to get in. "Come to my office" he said. So, he twisted my recalcitrant arm, application was made, and on my 18th birthday I sat the first of the Cambridge Entrance Exams. A couple of weeks later I went to Cambridge, to Trinity College, for interview, and here luck struck again, as I met Pat Merton (1920–1999). Although I knew none of this at the time, Pat had qualified in medicine but did not practice, his career was in human physiology, working in Arnold Carmichael's MRC group at Queen Square and in the Cambridge Physiological Laboratory. I remember little about our interview, other than the fact that we somehow got on to the subject of George Henry Lewes, someone I had at least heard of, specifically as the partner of the author Marian Evans, better known by her pseudonym of George Eliot, some of whose novels I had read (my sister around that time had worked as a nurse at the George Eliot Hospital in Nuneaton). Presumably Pat must have detected some kind of potential, worth taking a chance on (or maybe there was a quota of non-public school candidates to be fulfilled?), but the next thing I knew was, on Christmas Eve, the headmaster was knocking at the door of our house and saying "Congratulations, Andrew, you got a place at Cambridge". I later discovered the reason for this unprecedented visit: There were apparently concerns at the school, which at most got one or two pupils into Oxbridge each year, that I would turn down the offer of a place because of – get this, you will never believe it – because of my "bolshy" nature!

Well, I took the place, I went to Cambridge, and of course, I was a fish out of water, I didn't know what I was doing. (It might be argued that I have never known what I was doing ever since.) I was lucky that Roger Keynes was my Director of Studies at Trinity, so kept me on the straight and narrow, and he also afforded me, in my final year, my first opportunity to undertake some research in his lab. From him I learned a key lesson: one must at least try to make a contribution, and this aspiration has stayed with me and has been one of the drivers of my subsequent attempts at work (as opposed to my occupation).

One of the joys, privileges of medical education is the chance to learn human anatomy; at this time in Cambridge it was through hands-on cadaveric dissection, to which end, after our introductory lecture, we were instructed to line up in pairs and file into the dissecting room to be assigned our cadaver. But I had no "pair", so my plan was to declare this on reaching the front of the queue in the anticipation that there must be at least one other student in the same predicament. But before that happened, someone tapped me on the shoulder and said "Andrew, shall we dissect together?". And this despite the fact that he had been warned, by some of our contemporaries, that I was a "bit odd". So I don't know if it was bravery, desperation, or a bit of both that prompted you, Crispin, but that was surely one of my luckiest liminal moments, since over the dissecting table we subsequently bonded, became great friends and have remained so for over 40 years, during which time I came to know your late parents, your brothers, your wife, your children (to one of whom I am godfather) and now your grandchildren. So I have done very well out of the friendship; what's been in it for you is less clear to me, but that's a thread I don't presume to tug at too vigorously!

So, I struggled through Cambridge, and was then lucky enough to get a place at the Clinical School at the "other place", where luck strikes again. In the initial assignments students were organised alphabetically, and as L is next to M, I met Michael Mansfield. Being the efficient guy he is, Mike had already teamed up with Sally, so I have never known them other than as a couple, and we have been great friends now for almost 40 years.

After Oxford, and qualification, it was the journeyman existence of the junior medic, which took me to Birmingham, Oxford, London, Newcastle, the West Midlands, Cambridge (for my doctorate in Roger Keynes's lab), London again, and finally to Liverpool. It was demanding work but one of the consolations when progressing through the training grades was meeting other junior doctors who became friends. Over a brief period in the late 1990s I was lucky enough to meet three outstanding individuals: Parashkev Nachev when he was a medical student at Cambridge; Alex Leff when he was an SHO at Queen Square; and Miratul Muqit when he was an SHO at Charing Cross. All have gone on to achieve incredible things in neurology and neuroscience. Of course, they would have achieved all these things without ever meeting me, but I like to indulge myself with the thought that perhaps some occasional advice or direction, or an early shared publication, might have given them a little assistance early in their careers.

That is something I tried to continue throughout the Liverpool years, entirely informally. Although I think I was, technically at least, an "Educational Supervisor" or "Clinical Supervisor", or even both at some times, I had no idea what these bureaucratic terms meant or required. Here is a list of those Liverpool neurology Registrars that I have published at least one abstract or paper with; ditto Liverpool neurology Consultants; and external collaborators.

What do these publications add up to? Not much. A summation of "What I did" would quickly evaporate in any reader's mind: no one big thing, but perhaps many minuscule things (although hopefully done in a scholarly manner). I devoted much time to the now much despised genre of case reports, believing that they represent in some way the idiom of clinical practice. However, the works to which I devoted most time over more than 20 years were the pragmatic studies of cognitive and other screening instruments, but I now judge this work in particular to have been essentially a dead end, of its time, unenduring other than possibly as a historical curio. If it is true that Science is provisional, then so much more must that be the case for an inexact science like clinical medicine. If science, that is medical science, is not merely cultural relativism, but is progressive – as I believe it is – then it is to be expected that the outcome should be that "I have failed after many seasons/To bring truth to birth".

So, how to conclude? Whether one is thinking of the spoken word or of the written word, eventually one must come to the Bard. (Hence I top and tail my talk with Montaigne and Shakespeare, related writers.) The literary critic Harold Bloom found a "pragmatic nihilism" in the plays, and his description of Shakespeare suggests that he was, and is, cognitively beyond us, a form of words which simultaneously and paradoxically I do not understand but am in agreement with. I presume it means that Shakespeare took something common to us all, the faculty of language, and did with it what no one else can, in ways which are aesthetically and cognitively engaging and challenging, not only to his own time but in perpetuity. There are many quotations with which I might finish, but I choose the one which speaks to me most deeply. Of course, I have no idea how these lines should be delivered, being no orator, far less an actor, and I cannot read the whole solilioquy for fear of collapsing under its emotional weight. But I think this is the supreme Socratic moment of the life examined, and hence an appropriate summary for this career, and most particularly for this talk. I think it goes something like this:

> a poor player,
> That struts and frets his hour upon the stage,
> And then is heard no more. It is a tale
> Told by an idiot, full of sound and fury,
> Signifying nothing.
>
> (*Macbeth* V.v.19–28)

Acknowledgement

This is the substance (not transcript) of an address delivered at the Liverpool Medical Institution, 18th April 2024. Unpublished (and unpublishable!).

Reference

1.   Screech MA (ed.). *Michel de Montaigne. The complete Essays*. London: Penguin, 1991:40. [Other translations render this passage differently.]

Index